Horse Anatomy Coloring Book

1
2
3
4
5
6
7
8
9
10
11
12
13

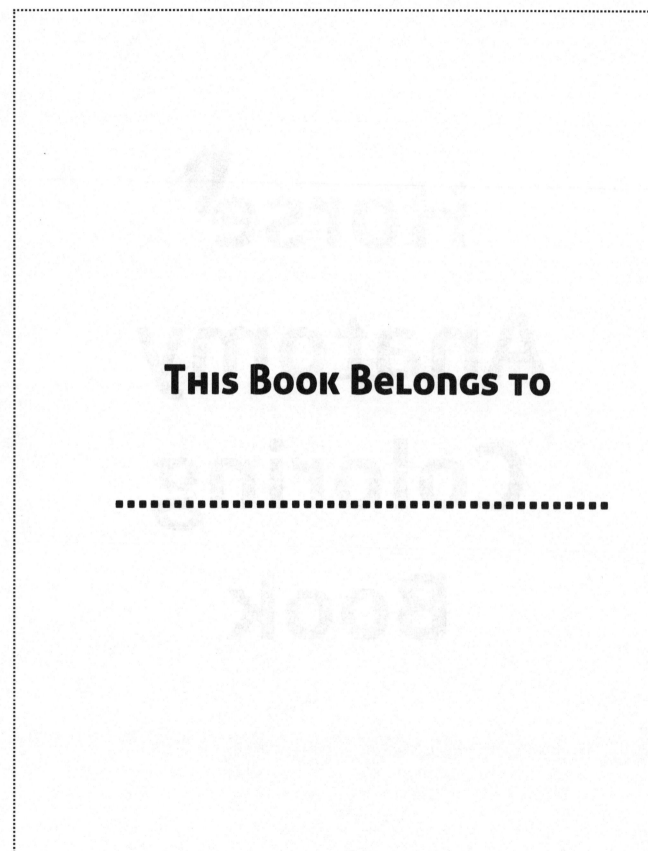

THIS BOOK BELONGS TO

....

Horse Skeleton (Lateral View)

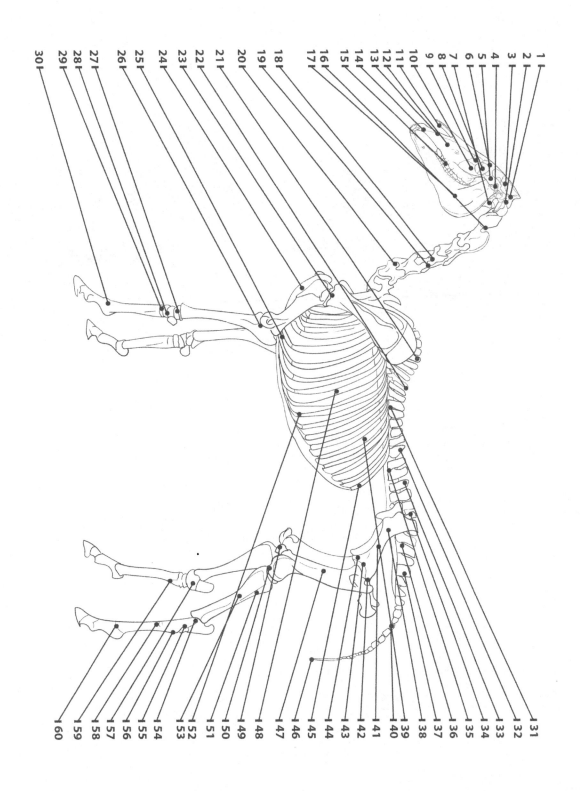

Horse Skeleton (Lateral View)

1. Occipital bone
2. Atiantooccipital joint
3. Parietal bone
4. Temporomandibuiar joint
5. Zygomatic arch
6. Frontal bone
7. Hyoid apparatus [Hyoid bone]
8. orbit
9. Lacrimal bone
10. Zygomatic bone
11. Nasal bone
12. Maxilla
13. Nasal process of incisive bone
14. Incisive bone
15. Teetn
16. Atlantoaxial joint
17. Mandible
18. Cervical vertebrae
19. Joints of articular processes
20. Intervertebral symphysis
21. Spinous process
22. Thoracic vertebrae
23. Shoulder joint
24. Sternum
25. Stemocostal joints
26. Elbow joint
27. Antebrachiocarpal joint
28. Carpal joints
29. Carpometacarpal joint
30. Metacarpophalangeal joints
31. Costovertebral joints
32. T18
33. Lumbar vertebrae
34. L6
35. Vertebral column
36. Sacrum [Sacral vertebrae]
37. S5
38. Ilium
39. Ribs
40. Caudal vertebrae [Coccygeal]
41. Coxal bone
42. Ischium
43. Hip joint
44. Pubis
45. Rib- 18
46. Cd 18
47. Thigh bone [Femur]
48. Thoracic cavity
49. Patella
50. Stifle joint
51. Fibula
52. Costochondral joints
53. Tibia
54. Tarsal joint
55. Tarsal bones
56. Metatarsal IV
57. Intertarsal joints
58. Metatarsal III
59. Metatarsal I
60. Metatarsophalangeal joints

Horse Skeleton (Cranial View)

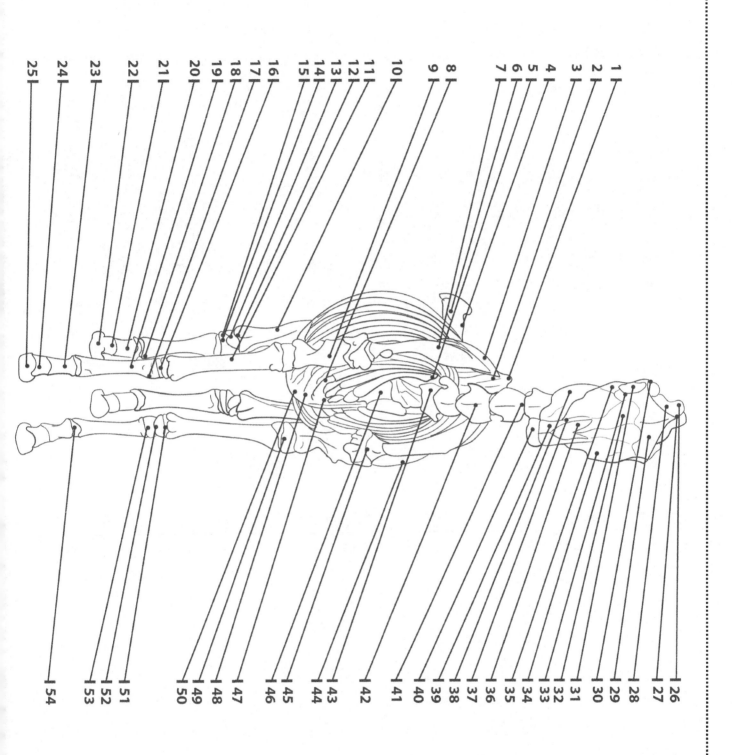

Horse Skeleton (Cranial View)

1. Spinous process
2. Thoracic vertebrae
3. Cartilage of scapula
4. Iliac crest
5. Costovertebral joints
6. Ilium
7. Scapula
8. Costal cartiage
9. Humerus
10. Tibia
11. Radius
12. Tarsocrural joint
13. Talus
14. Tarsal bones
15. Intertarsal joints
16. Carpal bones
17. Metacarpal II
18. Metacarpal IV
19. Metacarpal III
20. Proximal phalanx [Long pastern bone]
21. Middle phalanx [Short pastern bone]
22. Distal phalanx [Ungual bone, Coffin bone, Pedal bone]
23. Proximal phalanx [Long pastern bone]
24. Middle phalanx [Short pastern bone]
25. Distal phalanx [Ungual bone, Coffin bone, Pedal bone]
26. Occpital bone
27. External sagittal crest (Parietal bone)
28. Parietal bone
29. Frontal bone
30. Zygomatic arch
31. Orbit
32. Nasal bone
33. Lacrimal bone
34. Maxilla
35. Zygomatic bone
36. Nasal cavity
37. Nasal process of incisive bone
38. Mandible
39. Incisive bone
40. Teeth
41. Intervertebral symphysis
42. Cenvical vertebrae
43. Vertebral column
44. Ribs
45. Shoulder joint
46. Thoracic cavity
47. Sternal synchondroses
48. Sternocostal joints
49. Elbow joint
50. Sternum
51. Antebrachiocarpal joint
52. Carpal joints
53. Carpometacarpal joints
54. Metacarpophalangeal joints

Horse Skeleton (Caudal View)

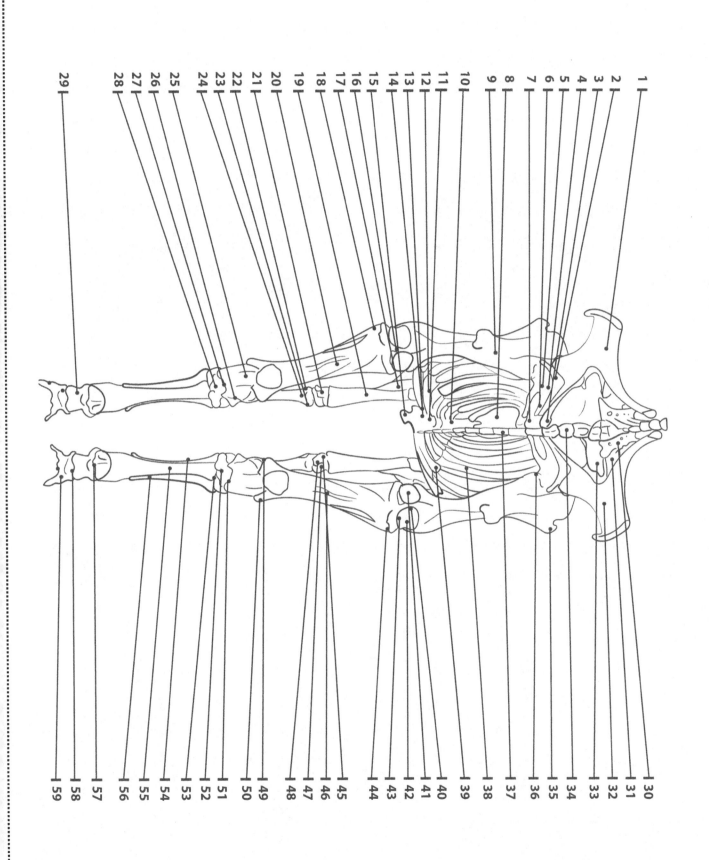

Horse Skeleton (Caudal View)

1. Ilium
2. Ischial arch
3. Ischial tuberosity
4. Ischiatic table
5. Ischium
6. Obturator foramen
7. Pubis
8. Thoracic cavity
9. Thigh bone [Femur]
10. Sternebrae
11. Sternum
12. Costal cartilage
13. Sternocostal joints
14. Steral synchondroses
15. Xiphoid process
16. Stifle joint
17. Ulna
18. Fibula
19. Radius
20. Tibia
21. Accessory carpal bone [Pisiform]|
22. Metacarpal IV
23. Metacarpal II
24. Metacarpal III
25. Calcaneus
26. Talus
27. Tarsal joint
28. Tarsal bones
29. Proximal phalanx[Long pastern bone]
30. Sacrum [Sacral vertebrae]
31. Sacroiliac joint
32. Coxal bone
33. Lumbar vertebrae
34. Caudal vertebrae [Coccygeal]
35. Greater trochanter
36. Hip joint
37. Vertebral column
38. Ribs
39. Costochondral joints
40. Intercondylar fossa
41. Medial condyle
42. Lateral condyle
43. Femorotibial joint
44. Head of fibula
45. Antebrachiocarpal joint
46. Body [Shaft] of tibia
47. Carpal joints
48. Carpal bones
49. Medial malleolus
50. Lateral malleolus
51. Tarsocrural joint
52. Intertarsal joints
53. Tarsometatarsal joints
54. Metatarsal II
55. Metatarsal III
56. Metatarsal IV
57. Metatarsophalangeal joints
58. Proximal interphalangeal joint
59. Distal interphalangeal joint

Horse Skeleton (Dorsal View)

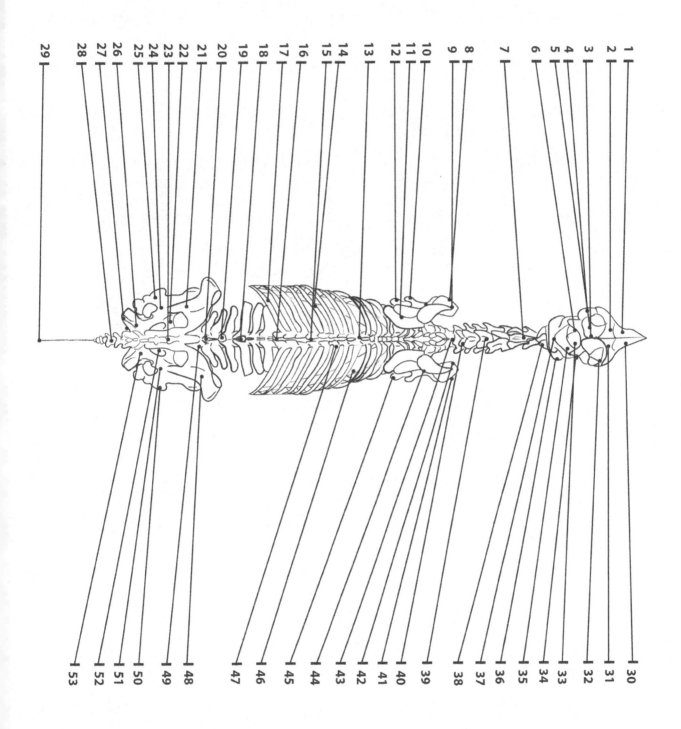

Horse Skeleton (Dorsal View)

1. Maxila
2. Forehead
3. External sagittal crest [Parietal bone]
4. Parietal bone
5. Temporomandibular joint
6. Occiput
7. Axis
8. Shoulder joint
9. Humerus
10. Lateral epicondyle
11. Cartilage of scapula
12. Ulna
13. Thoracic vertebrae
14. Spinous process
15. Ribs
16. T18
17. Rib -18
18. Lumbar vertebrae
19. Vertebral column
20. L6
21. Coxal bone
22. Pubis
23. Sacrum [Sacral vertebrae]
24. Hip joint
25. Thigh bone [Femur]
26. Ischium
27. Ischial tuberosity
28. Caudal vertebrae [Coccygeal]
29. Cd 18
30. Nasal bone
31. Frontal bone
32. Zygomatic arch
33. Mandible
34. Occipital bone
35. Atlantooccipital joint
36. Transverse process [Atlantal wing]
37. Atlas
38. Atlantoaxial joint
39. Cervical vertebrae
40. Joints of articular processes
41. Greater tubercle
42. Lesser tubercle
43. C7
44. Scapula
45. Olecranon tuber
46. Thoracic cavity
47. Costovertebral joints
48. Ilium
49. Lumbosacral joints
50. Greater trochanter
51. Acetabulum
52. Obturator foramen
53. Ischiatic table

Horse - Cranium (Lateral view)

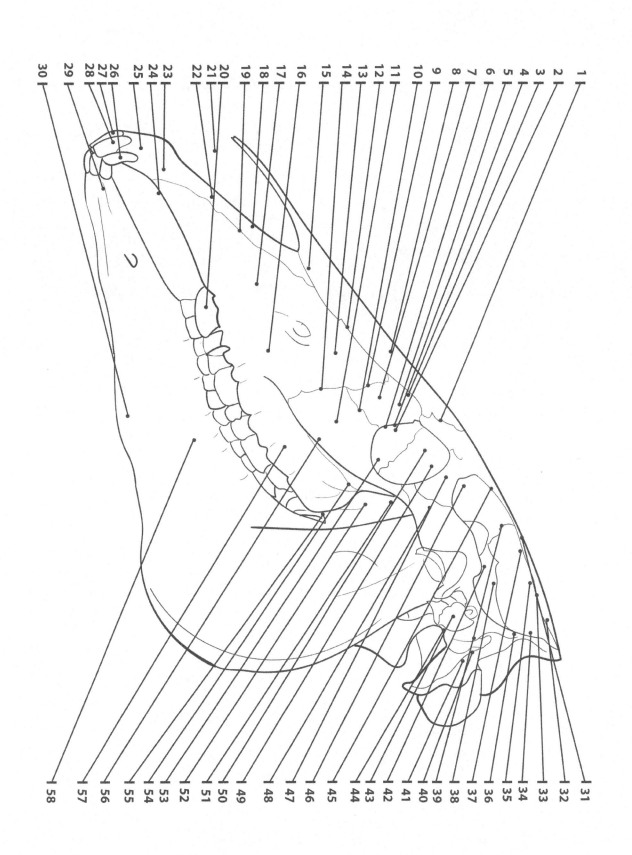

Horse - Cranium (Lateral view)

1. Frontonasal suture
2. Orbital surface of lacrimal bone
3. Nasolacrimal suture
4. Fossa for lacrimal sac
5. Lacrimal bone
6. Lacrimal foramen
7. Facial surface of lacrimal bone
8. Nasal bone
9. Lacrimomaxillary suture
10. Lacrimozygomatic suture
11. Lateral surface of zygomatic bone
12. Nasomaxillary suture
13. Facial surface of maxilla
14. Zygomaticomaxillary suture
15. Nasoincisive suture
16. Body of maxilla
17. Maxilla
18. Nasal process of incisive bone
19. Maxilloincisive suture
20. First premolar
21. Osseous nasal aperture
22. Incisive bone
23. Body of incisive bone
24. Canine tooth
25. Alveolar process of incisive bone
26. Third incisor
27. First incisor
28. Second incisor
29. Incisive part of body of mandible
30. Body of mandible
31. External Sagittal Crest (parietal bone)
32. Occipitointerparietal suture
33. External sagittal crest (interparietal bone)
34. Lambdoid suture
35. Temporal line (inerparietal bone)
36. Occipitosquamous suture
37. Temporal line (Parietal bone)
38. Squamous suture
39. Coronal suture
40. Occipitomastoid suture
41. Lateral part of occipital bone
42. Squamous part of temporal bone
43. Tympanic part of temporal bone
44. Petrous part of temporal bone
45. Temporal line (Frontal bone)
46. Temporal surface of frontal bone
47. zygomatic process of frontal bone
48. Zagomatic proces of temporal bone
49. Orbital part of frontal bone
50. Orbital surface of frontal bone
51. Wing of presphenoid bone
52. Sphenopalatine suture
53. Orbital surface of zygomatic bone
54. Zygomatic process of maxilla
55. Pterygosphenoidalae suture
56. Facial crest of zygomatic bone
57. Alveolar process of maxilla
58. Molar part of body of mandible

Horse Cranium (Lateral View)

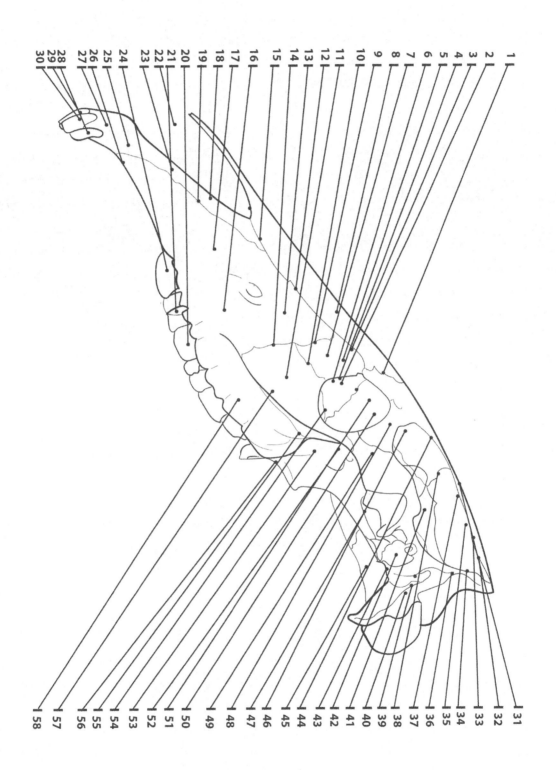

Horse Cranium (Lateral View)

1. Frontonasal suture
2. Orbital surface of lacrimal bone
3. Nasolacrimal suture
4. Fossa for lacrimal sac
5. Lacrimal bone
6. Lacrimal foramen
7. Facial surface of lacrimal bone
8. Nasal bone
9. Lacrimomaxillary suture
10. Lacrimozygomatic suture
11. Lateral surface of zygomatic bone
12. Nasomaxillary suture
13. Facial surface of maxilla
14. Zygomaticomaxillary suture
15. Nasoincisive suture
16. Body of maxilla
17. Maxilla
18. Nasal process of incisive bone
19. Maxilloincisive suture
20. First premolar
21. Osseous nasal aperture
22. Incisive bone
23. Body of incisive bone
24. Canine tooth
25. Alveolar process of incisive bone
26. Third incisor
27. First incisor
28. Second incisor
29. Incisive part of body of mandible
30. Body of mandible
31. Eternal sagittal crest (Parietal bone)
32. Occipitointerparietal suture
33. External sagittal crest (Interparietal bone)
34. Lambdoid suture
35. Temporal line (Interparietal bone)
36. Occipitosquamous suture
37. Temporal line (Parietal bone)
38. Coronal suture
39. Occipitomastoid suture
40. Lateral part of occipital bone
41. Squamous part of temporal bone
42. Tympanic part of temporal bone
43. Petrous part of temporal bone
44. Temporal line (Frontal bone)
45. Basilar part of occipital bone
46. Temporal surface of frontal bone
47. Sphenosquamous structure
48. zygomatic process of frontal bone
49. zygemate process of temporal bone
50. Orbital part of frontal bone
51. Orbital surface of frontal bone
52. Wing of presphenoid bone
53. Sphenopalatine suture
54. Orbital surface of zygomatic bone
55. Zygomatic process of maxila
56. Prerygosphenoicalae suture
57. Facial crest of zygomatic bone
58. Alveolar process of maxila

Horse - Cranium (Rostral view)

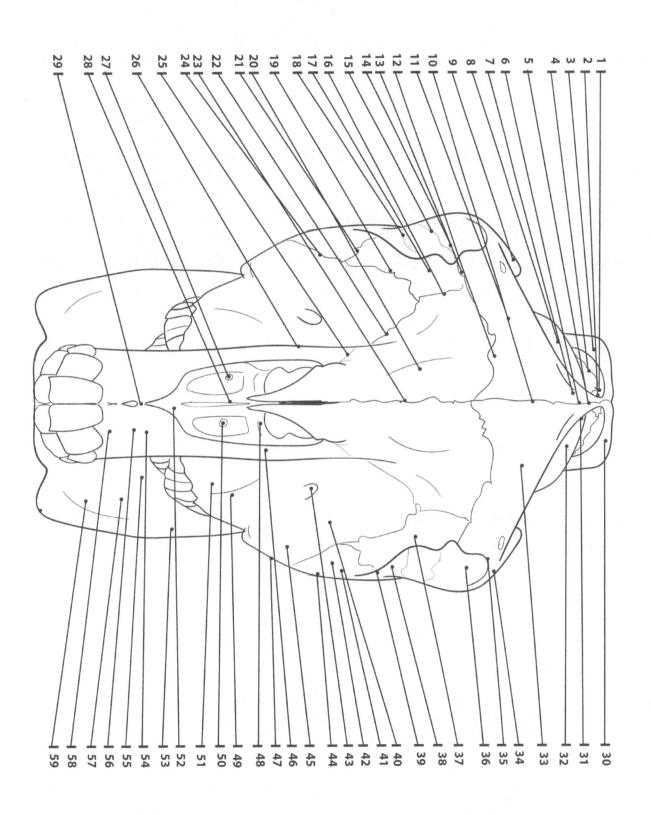

Horse - Cranium (Rostral view)

1. Occipitointerparietal suture
2. Interarietal bone
3. Occiptal bone
4. Lambdoid suture
5. Exteral sagittal crest (Parieta bone)
6. Sagittal suture
7. Coronal suture
8. Parietal bone
9. Zygomatic arch
10. Interfrontal suture
11. Frontal bone
12. Frontonasal suture
13. Frontolacrimal suture
14. Orbit
15. Frontozygomatic suture
16. Nasolacrimal suture
17. Lacrimal bone
18. Temporozygomatic suture
19. Lacrimomaxillary suture
20. Nasal bone
21. Lacrimozygomatic suture
22. Nasomaxillary suture
23. Internasal suture
24. Zygomaticomaxillary suture
25. Nasoincisive suture
26. Maxilloincisive suture
27. Nasal cavity
28. Vomer
29. Interincisive suture
30. Nuchal crest
31. Temporal line (Parietal bone)
32. Parietal tuberositiy
33. Squamous part of frontal bone
34. Zygomatic process of frontal bone
35. Supraorbital margin
36. Orbital part of frontal bone
37. Facial surface of lacrimal bone
38. Orvbital surface of zygomatic bone
39. infraorbital margin
40. Facial surface of maxilla
41. Lateral surface of zygomatic bone
42. Zygomatic bone
43. infraorbital foramen
44. Facial crest of zygomatic bone
45. Body of maxilla
46. Nasal process of incisive bone
47. Facial crest
48. Horizontal plate of palatine bone
49. Alveolar process of maxilla
50. Palatine process (Maxilla)
51. Alveolar yokes
52. Palatine process of incisive bone
53. Ramus of mandible
54. Body of incisive bone
55. Molar part of body of mandible
56. Labial surface
57. Body of mandible
58. Alveolar process of incisive bone
59. Buccal surface

Horse - Cranium (Rostral view)

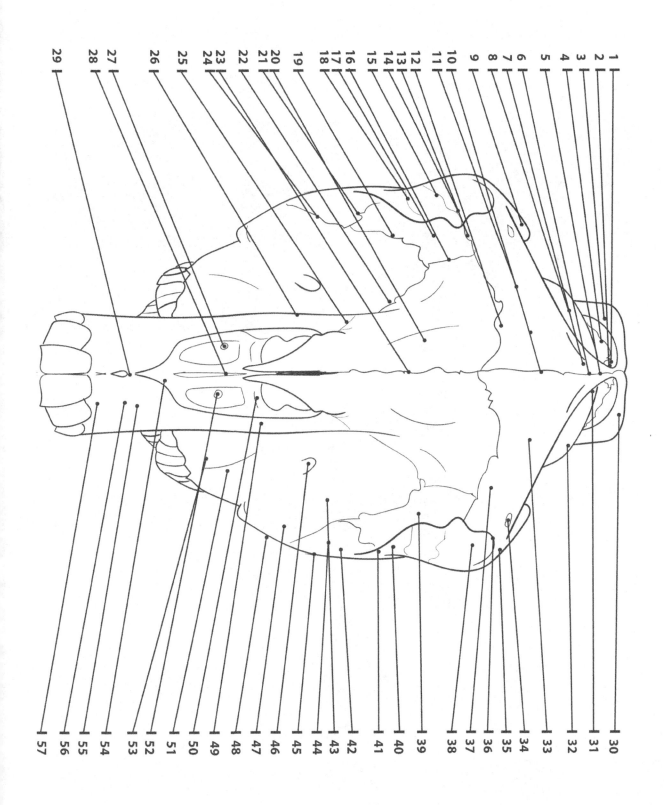

Horse-Cranium (Rostral view)

1. Occipitointerparital suture
2. Inerparietal bone
3. Occiptal bone
4. Lambdoid suture
5. Extemal sagittal crest(Parital bone)
6. Sagittal suture
7. Coronal suture
8. Parietal bone
9. Zygomatic arch
10. Interfrontal suture
11. Frontal bone
12. Frontonasal suture
13. Frontolacrimal suture
14. Orbit
15. Frontozygomatic suture
16. Nasolacrimal suture
17. Lacrimal bone
18. Temporozygomatic suture
19. Lacrimomaxillary suture
20. Nasal bone
21. Lacrimozygomtic suture
22. Nasomaxillary suture
23. Intenasal suture
24. Zygomaticomaxillary suture
25. Nasoincisive suture
26. Maxilloincisive suture
27. Nasal cavity
28. Vomer
29. Interincisive suture
30. Nuchal crest
31. Temporal line (Parietal bone)
32. Parital tuberositiy
33. Sauamous part of fontal bone
34. Supraorbital foramen
35. Zygomtic process of frotal bone
36. Supraorbital margin
37. Frontal tuberositiy
38. Orbital part of frontal bone
39. Facial surface of lacrimal bone
40. Orbital surface of zygomatic bone
41. Infraorbital margin
42. Lateral surface of zygomatic bone
43. Facial surface of maxilla
44. Zygomatic bone
45. Facil crest of zygomatic bone
46. Infraorbital foramen
47. Body of maxilla
48. Facial crest
49. Nasal procsss of incisive bone
50. Horizontal plate of palatine bone
51. Alveolar process of maxilla
52. Palatine process (Maxilla)
53. Aevolar yokes
54. Palatine process of incisive bone
55. Booy of incisive bone
56. Labial surface
57. Alveolar process of incisive bone

Horse - Cranium (Caudal view)

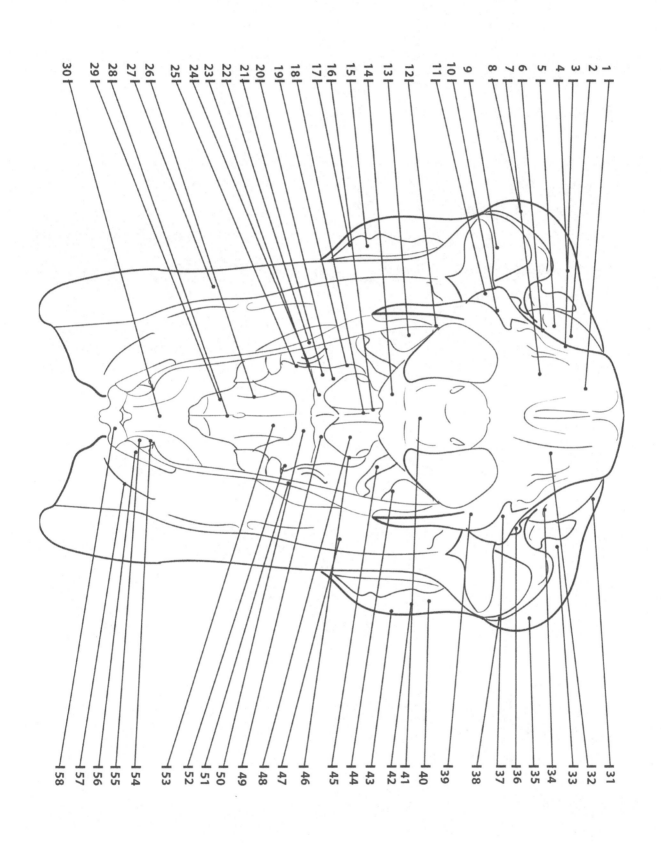

Horse - Cranium (Caudal view)

1. Occiput
2. Parietal bone
3. Lambdoid suture
4. Frontal bone
5. Squamous suture
6. Occipitosquamous suture
7. Occipital bone
8. .Zygomatic arch
9. Temporomandibular oint
10. Occipitomastoid suture
11. 'Squamomastoidsous suture
12. Temporohyoid joint
13. Plerygopalatine fossa
14. Basisphenoid bone
15. Mavila
16. Vomer
17. Zygomaticomaxilary suture
18. Bony nasal septum
19. Sphenopalatine suture
20. Nasal cavity
21. Palatine bone
22. Hyoid apparatus [Hyoid bone]
23. Bony palate
24. Plerygosphenoidalae suture
25. Plerygoid bone
26. Palatine fissure
27. Mandible
28. Interincisive canal
29. Incisive bone
30. Intermandibutar joint
31. Temporal line (Frontal bone)
32. Squamous part of occipial bone
33. Temporal surface of frontal bone
34. Squamous part of temporal bone
35. Zygomatic process of frontal bone
36. Tympanic part of temporal bone
37. Petrous part of temporal bone
38. Zygomatic process of temporal bone
39. Lateral part of occipital bone
40. Temporal process
41. Basilar part of occipital bone
42. Zygomatic bone
43. Facial crest of zygomatic bone
44. Caudal palatine foramen
45. Pterygoid process
46. Perpendicular plate of palatine bone
47. Ramus of mandible
48. Choanae
49. Horizontal plate of palatine bone
50. Palatine process(Maxilla)
51. Stylohyoid
52. Pterygoid hamulus
53. Palatine process of incisive bone
54. Epihyoid
55. Ceratohyoid (Lesser horn)
56. Thyrohyoid (Great horn)
57. Body of mandible
58. Basinyoid [Body]

Horse - Cranium (Caudal view)

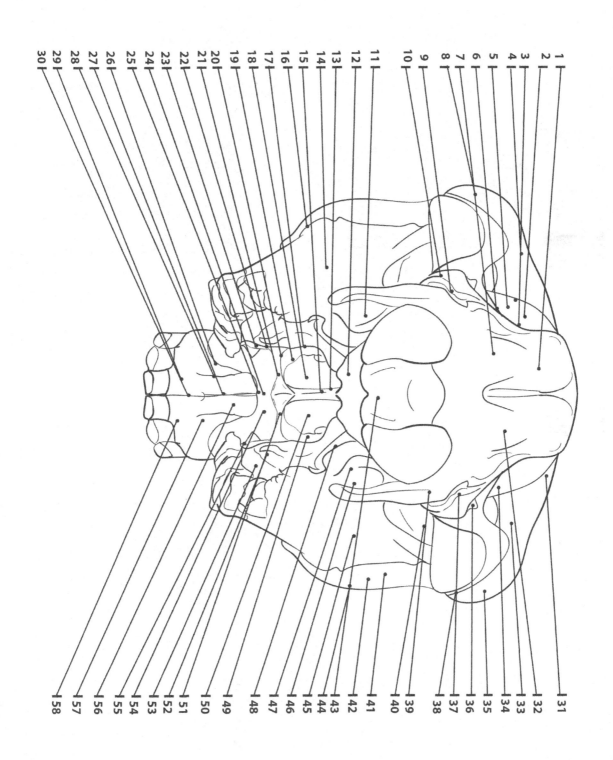

Horse - Cranium (Caudal view)

1. Occiput
2. Parietal bone
3. Lambdoid suture
4. Frontal bone
5. Squamous suture
6. Occipitosquamous suture
7. Occipital bone
8. Zygomatic arch
9. Occipitomastoid suture
10. Squamomastoideous suture
11. Pterygopalatine fossa
12. Basisphenoid bone
13. Vomer
14. Maxilla
15. Bony nasal septum
16. Zygomaticomaxillary suture
17. Sphenopalatine suture
18. Osseous nasal aperture
19. Nasal cavity
20. Palatine bone
21. Bony palate
22. Pterygosphenoidalae suture
23. Pterygoid bone
24. Torus palatinus
25. Median palatine suture
26. Maxilloincisive suture
27. Interincisive suture
28. Palatine fissure
29. Interincisive canal
30. Incisive bone
31. Temporal line (Frontal bone)
32. Squamous part of occipial bone
33. Temporal surface of frontal bone
34. Squamous partof temporal bone
35. Zygomatic process of fontal bone
36. Tympanic part of temporal bone
37. Petrous part of temporal bone
38. Zygometic process of temporal bone
39. Latera part of occipital bone
40. Orbital surface of zygomatic bone
41. Temporal process
42. Zygomatic bone
43. Basilar part of occipital bone
44. Facial rest of zygomatic bone.
45. Bodyy of maxilla
46. Pterygopalatine surface of maxilla
47. Caudal palatine foramen
48. Pterygoid process
49. Perpendicular plate of palatine bone
50. Choanae
51. Horizontal plate of palatine bone
52. Palatine groove
53. Alveolar process of maxilla
54. Palatine process (Maxilla)
55. Plerygoid hamulus
56. Palatine process of incisive bone
57. Body of incisive bone
58. Alveolar process of incsive bone

Horse Cranium (Dorsal View

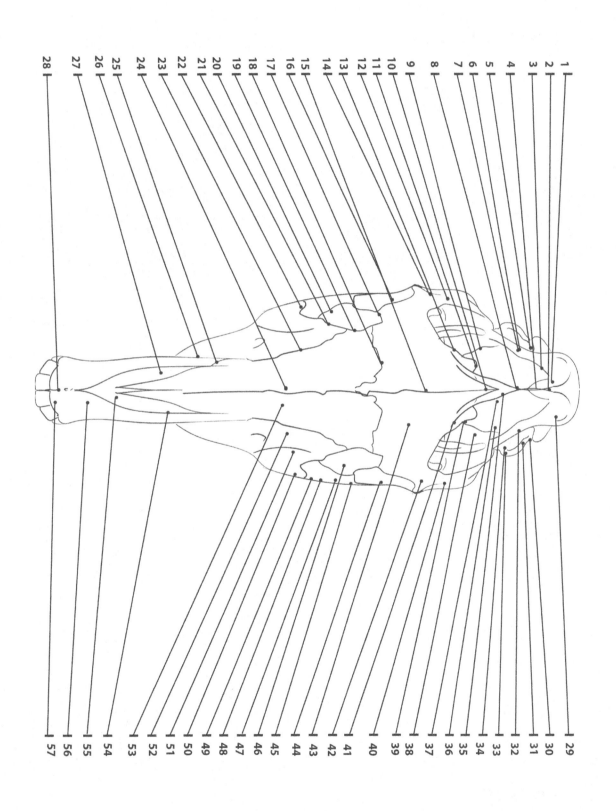

Horse Cranium (Dorsal View)

1. Occipitointerparietal suture
2. Temporal line (Interparietal bone)
3. Lambdoid suture
4. External sagittal crest (Interparietal bone)
5. Occipitomastoid suture
6. Occipitosquamous suture
7. Squamomastoideous suture
8. External sagittal crest (Parietal bone)
9. Squamous suture
10. Sagittal suture
11. Coronal suture
12. Zygomatic arch
13. Squaomosofrontal suture
14. Frontozygomatic suture
15. Interfrontal suture
16. Orbit
17. Frontolacrimal suture
18. Frontonasal suture
19. Nasolacrimal suture
20. Lacrimozygomatic suture
21. Lacrimomaxillary suture
22. Zygomaticomaxillary suture
23. Nasomaxillary suture
24. Internasal suture
25. Nasoincisive suture
26. Maxilloincisive suture
27. Nasal cavity
28. Interincisive suture
29. Nuchal crest
30. Petrous part of temporal bone
31. Mastoid process
32. Occipital process
33. External acoustic opening
34. Tympanic part of temporal bone
35. Temporal line (Parietal bone)
36. Temporal plane
37. Parietal plane
38. Squamous part of temporal bone
39. Temporal surface of frontal bone
40. Zygomatic process of temporal bone
41. Temporal line (Frontal bone)
42. Zygomatic process of frontal bone
43. Squamous part of frontal bone
44. Orbital surface of zygomatic bone
45. Infraorbital margin
46. Facial surface of lacrimal bone
47. Zygomatic bone
48. Lateral surface of zygomatic bone
49. Facial crest of zygomatic bone
50. Zygomatic process of maxilla
51. Facial surface of maxilla
52. Body of maxilla
53. Palatine process (Maxilla)
54. Nasal process of incisive bone
55. Palatine process of incisive bone
56. Body of incisive bone
57. Alveolar process of incisive bone

Horse - Cranium (Ventral view)

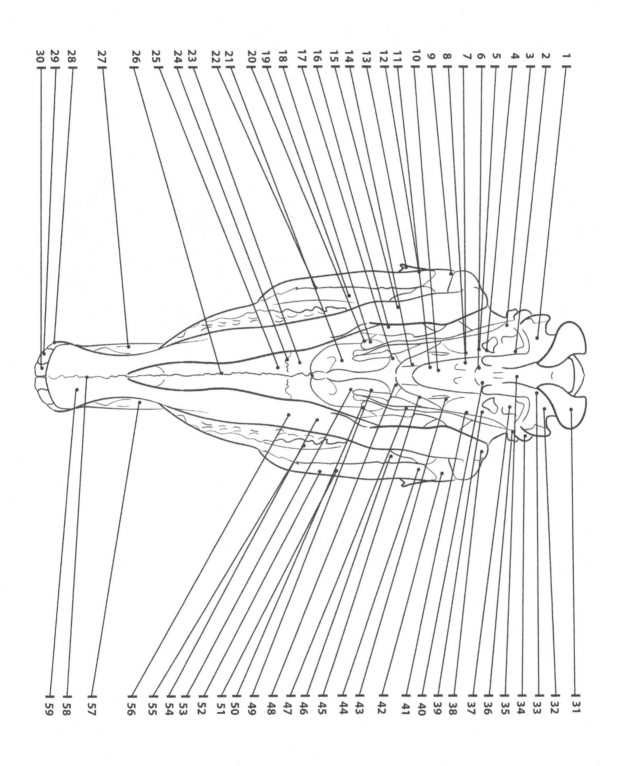

Horse - Cranium (Ventral view)

1. Occipital bone
2. Jugular foramen
3. Temporohyoid joint
4. Petrooccipital canal
5. Coronal suture
6. Sphenooccipital synchondrosis
7. Basisphenoid bone
8. Sphenosquamous suture
9. Temporomandibular joint
10. Intersphenoidal synchondrosis
11. Presphenoid bone
12. Temporozygomatic suture
13. Zygomatic arch
14. Vomerosphnoidal suture
15. Mandible
16. Pterygopalatine fossa
17. Hyoid apparatus [Hyoid bone]
18. Pterygoid bone
19. Maxilla
20. Pterygopalatine suture
21. Ethmoid bone
22. Zygomaticomaxillary suture
23. Palatine bone
24. Transverse palatine suture
25. Bony palate
26. Median palatine suture
27. Incisive bone
28. Third incisor
29. Second incisor
30. First incisor
31. Occipital condyle
32. Lateral part of occipital bone
33. Hypoglossal canal
34. Mastoid process
35. Basilar part of occipital bone
36. Tympanic part of temporal bone
37. Petrous part of temporal bone
38. Ramus of mandible
39. Muscular process
40. Muscular tubercle
41. Stylohyoid
42. Zygomatic process of temporal bone
43. Caudal alar foramen
44. Temporal process
45. Thyrohyoid [Great horn]
46. Zygomatic process of maxilla
47. Pterygoid process
48. Basihyoid [Body]
49. Ceratohyoid [Lesser horn]
50. Pterygoid hamulus
51. Zygomatic bone
52. Facial crest of zygomatic bone
53. Epihyoid
54. Molar part of body of mandible
55. Alveolar process of maxilla
56. Body of mandible
57. Nasal process of incisive bone
58. Intermandibular joint
59. Incisive part of body of mandible

Horse - Cranium (Ventral view)

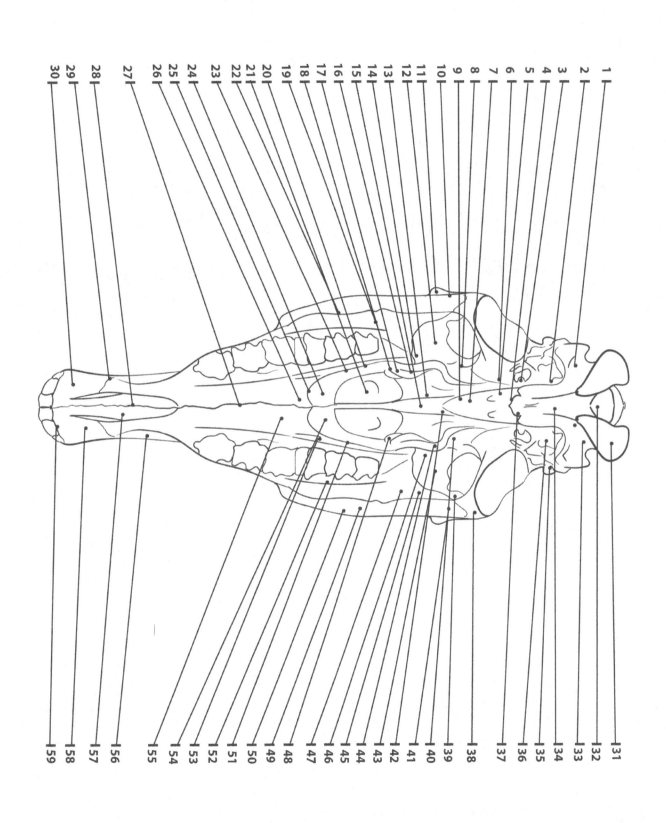

Horse - Cranium (Ventral view)

1. Occipital bone
2. Jugular foramen
3. Petrooccipital canal
4. Sphenooccipital synchondrosis
5. Basisphenoid bone
6. Sphenosquamous suture
7. Intersphenoidal synchondrosis
8. Presphenoid bone
9. Infratemporal fossa
10. Temporozygomatic suture
11. Zygomatic arch
12. Frontal bone
13. Vomerosphnoidal suture
14. Pterygopalatine fossa
15. Vomer
16. Pterygosphenoidalae suture
17. Pterygoid bone
18. Pterygopalatine suture
19. Maxilla
20. Palatomaxillary suture
21. Ethmoid bone
22. Zygomaticomaxillary suture
23. Greater palatine foramen
24. Palatine bone
25. Transverse palatine suture
26. Bony palate
27. Median palatine suture
28. Interincisive suture
29. Maxilloincisive suture
30. Incisive bone
31. Occipital condyle
32. Foramen magnum
33. Lateral part of occipital bone
34. Basilar part of occipital bone
35. Tympanic part of temporal bone
36. Petrous part of temporal bone
37. Muscular tubercle
38. Zygomatic process of temporal bone
39. Zygomatic process of frontal bone
40. Wing of presphenoid bone
41. Temporal process
42. Ala of vomer
43. Orbital part of frontal bone
44. Pterygoid process
45. Zygomatic process of maxilla
46. Orbital surface of frontal bone
47. Body of maxilla
48. Pterygoid hamulus
49. Zygomatic bone
50. Facial crest of zygomatic bone
51. Greater palatine foramen
52. Alveolar process of maxilla
53. Palatine groove
54. Horizontal plate of palatine bone
55. Palatine process (Maxilla)
56. Nasal process of incisive bone
57. Palatine process of incisive bone
58. Body of incisive bone
59. Alveolar process of incisive bone

Horse - Mandible (Craniolateral view)

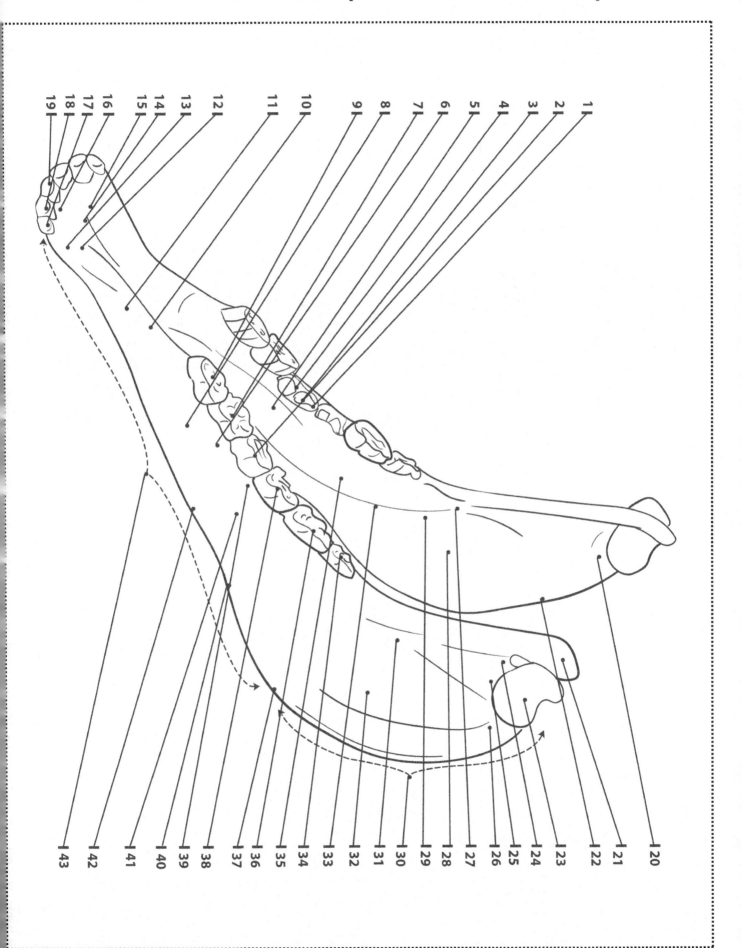

Horse - Mandible (Craniolateral view)

1. Interalveolar septa
2. Third premolar
3. Dental alveoli
4. Interradicular septa
5. Mylohyoid line
6. Alveolar yokes
7. Second premolar
8. Buccal surface
9. First premolar
10. Interalveolar border
11. Mental foramen
12. Canine tooth
13. Incisive part of body of mandible
14. Intermandibular joint
15. Labial surface
16. Alveolar arch
17. Third incisor
18. Second incisor
19. First incisor
20. Pterygoid fovea
21. Coronoid process
22. Sternomandibular muscle tuberosity
23. Head of mandible
24. Mandibular notch
25. Neck of mandible
26. Condylar process
27. Mandibular foramen
28. Pterygoid fossa
29. Mylohyoid groove
30. Ramus of mandible
31. Mandible
32. Masseteric fossa
33. Mandibular canal
34. Third molar tooth
35. Lingual surface
36. Second molar tooth
37. Angle of mandible
38. First molar tooth
39. Alveolar border
40. Notch for facial vessels
41. Molar part of body of mandible
42. Ventral border
43. Body of mandible

Horse - Mandible (Caudal view)

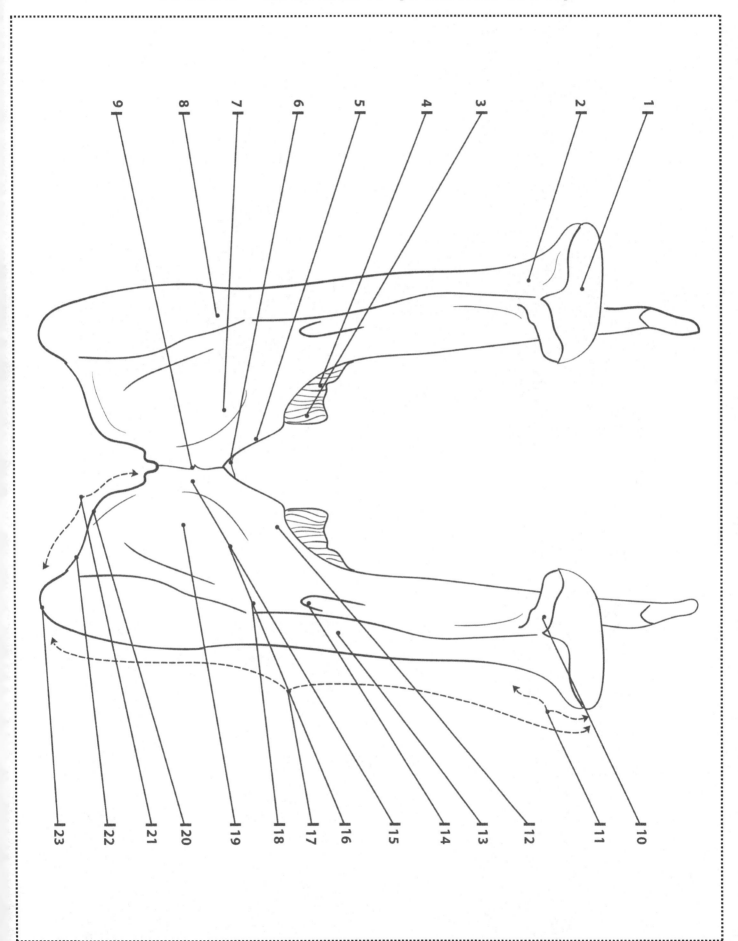

Horse - Mandible (Caudal view)

1. Head of mandible
2. Neck of mandible-
3. Premolar teeth
4. Molar teeth
5. Interalveolar border-
6. Incisors
7. Mylohyoid line
8. Mandible
9. Intermandibular joint
10. Pterygoid fovea
11. Condylar process
12. Alveolar border
13. Sternomandibular muscle tuberosity
14. Mandibular foramen
15. Incisive part of body of mandible
16. Molar part of body of
17. Ramus of mandible mandible
18. Mylohyoid groove
19. Lingual surface
20. Ventral border
21. Body of mandible
22. Notch for facial vessels
23. Angle of mandible

Horse - Hyoid apparatus (Craniolateral view)

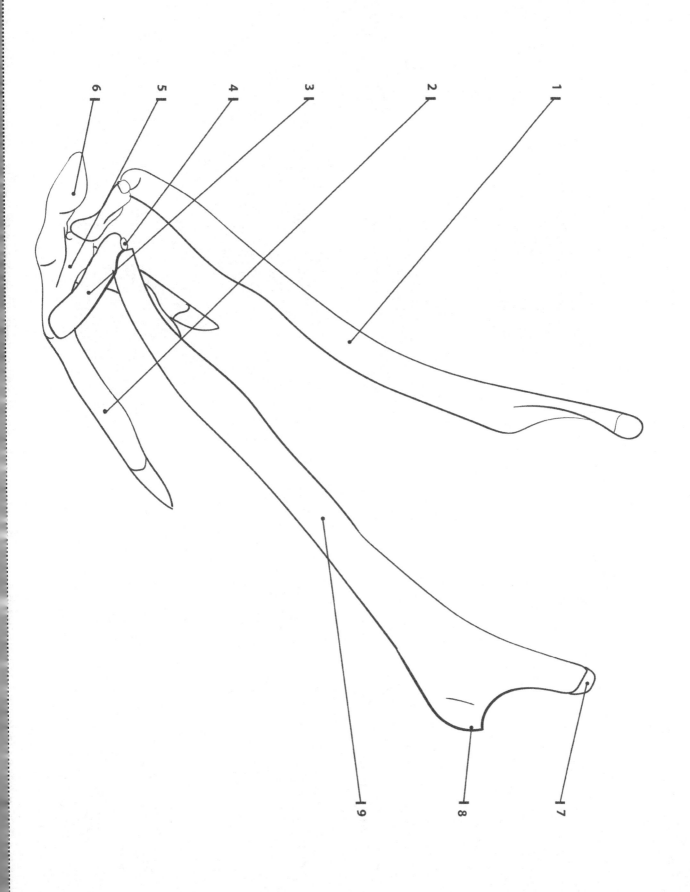

Horse - Hyoid apparatus (Craniolateral view)

1.Hyoid apparatus[Hyoid bone]
2.Thyrohyoid [Great horn]
3.Ceratohyoid [Lesser horn]
4.Epihyoid
5.Basihyoid [Body]
6.Lingual process

7.Tympanohyoid
8.Stylohyoid angle
9.Stylohyoid

Horse - Vertebral column (Lateral view)

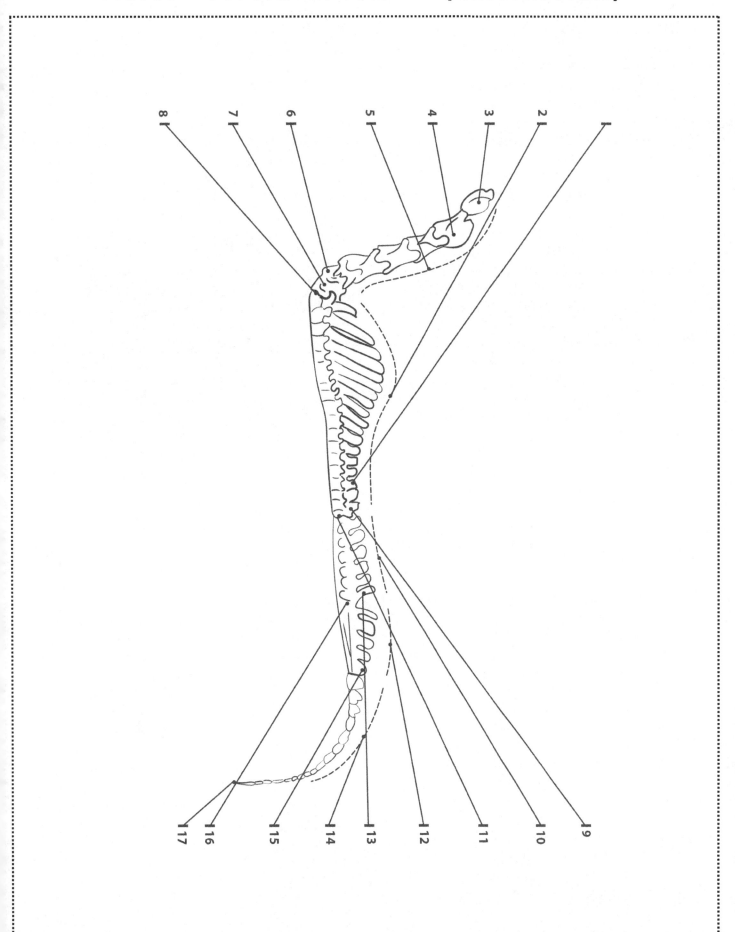

Horse - Vertebral column (Lateral view)

1. Anticlinal vertebra
2. Thoracic vertebrae
3. Atlas
4. Axis
5. Cervical vertebrae
6. Vertebral column
7. C7
8. Cervicothoracic vertebral junction
9. T18
10. Lumbar vefiebraei
11. Thoracolumbar vertebral junction
12. Sacrum Sacral vertebrae
13. L6
14. Caudal vertebrae [Coccygeal]
15. S5
16. Lumbosacral vertebral junction
17. Cd18

Horse - Vertebral column (Dorsal view)

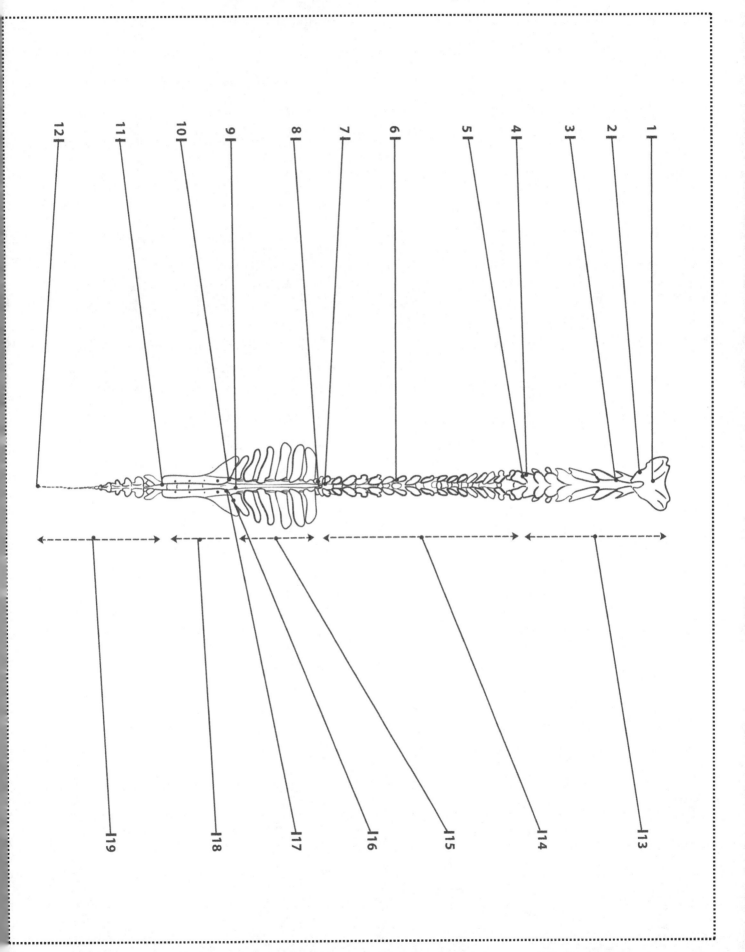

Horse - Vertebral column (Dorsal view)

1. Atlas
2. Atlantoaxial Joint
3. Axis
4. C7
5. Cervicothoracic vertebral junction
6. Vertebral column
7. T18
8. Thoracolumbar vertebral junction
9. L6
10. Lumbosacral vertebral junction
11. S5
12. Cd18

13. Cervical vertebrae
14. Thoracic vertebrae
15. Lumbar vertebrae
16. Lumbosacral intertransversar joint
17. Lumbosacral joint
18. Sacrum [Sacral vertebrae]
19. Caudal vertebrae[Coccygeal]

Horse - Cervical vertebrae (Lateral view)

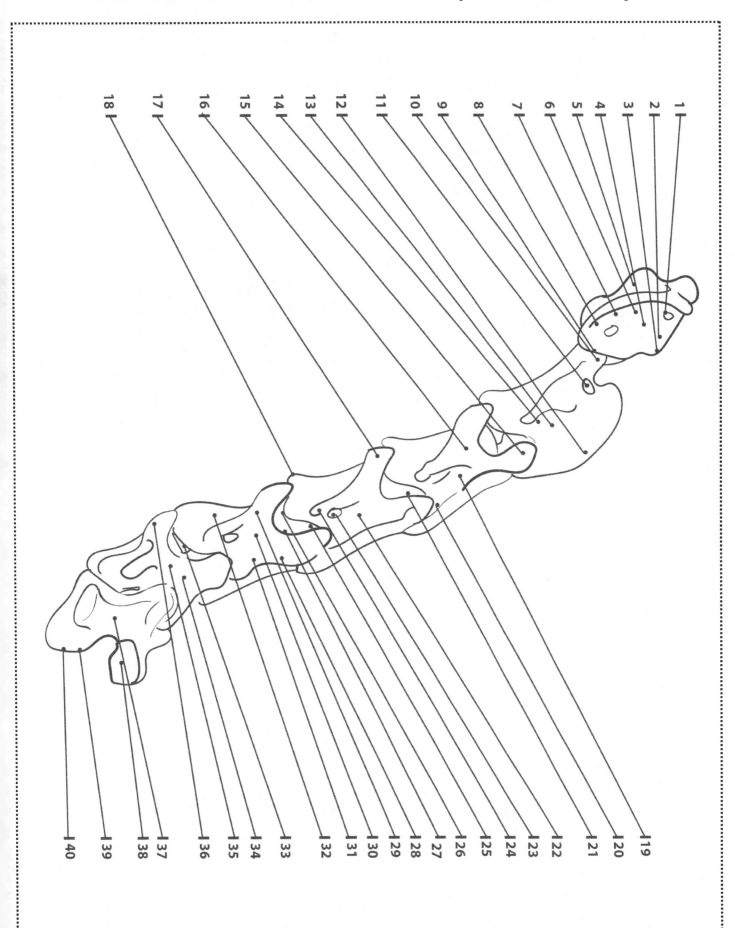

Horse - Cervical vertebrae (Lateral view)

1. Alar foramen
2. Dorsal arch
3. Dorsal tubercle
4. Lateral mass
5. Ventral arch
6. Atlas
7. C1
8. Transverse process [Atlantal wing]
9. Atlantoaxial joint
10. Dens
11. Lateral vertebral foramen
12. Spinous process
13. Axis
14. C2
15. Cranial articular process
16. Transverse process
17. Ventral tubercle
18. Ventral crest
19. C3
20. Joints of articular processes
21. Intervertebral foramen
22. C4
23. Transverse foramen
24. Dorsal tubercle
25. Caudal vertebral notch
26. Intervertebral symphysis
27. Cranial vertebral notch
28. Lamina of vertebral arch
29. Transverse process
30. C5
31. Vertebral arch
32. Vertebral body
33. Cranial extremity [Vertebral head]
34. C6
35. Pedicle of vertebral arch
36. Ventral plate [Cervical vertebra VI]
37. C7
38. Caudal articular process
39. Caudal costal fovea [Cervical vertebra C7]
40. Caudal extremity [Vertebral fossa]

Horse - Cervical vertebrae (Dorsal view)

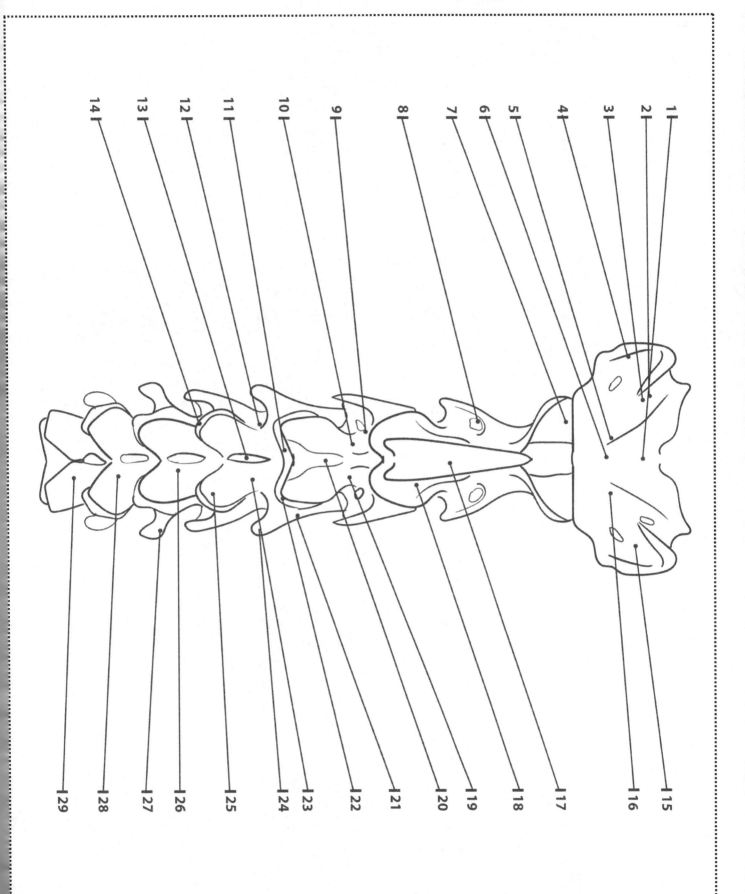

Horse - Cervical vertebrae (Dorsal view)

1. Atlas
2. Alar foramen
3. Lateral vertebral foramen
4. Transverse process [Atlantal wing]
5. Dorsal arch
6. Dorsal tubercle
7. Atlantoaxial joint
8. Transverse forament
9. Pedicle of vertebral arch
10. Lamina of vertebral arch
11. Interarcual space
12. Intervertebral foramen
13. Spinous process
14. Joints of articular processes
15. Lateral mass
16. C1
17. C2
18. Axis
19. Vertebral arch
20. C3
21. Transverse process
22. Cranial articular process
23. C4
24. Dorsal tubercle
25. Caudal articular process
26. C5
27. Transverse process
28. C6
29. C7

Horse - Atlas - C1 (Lateral view)

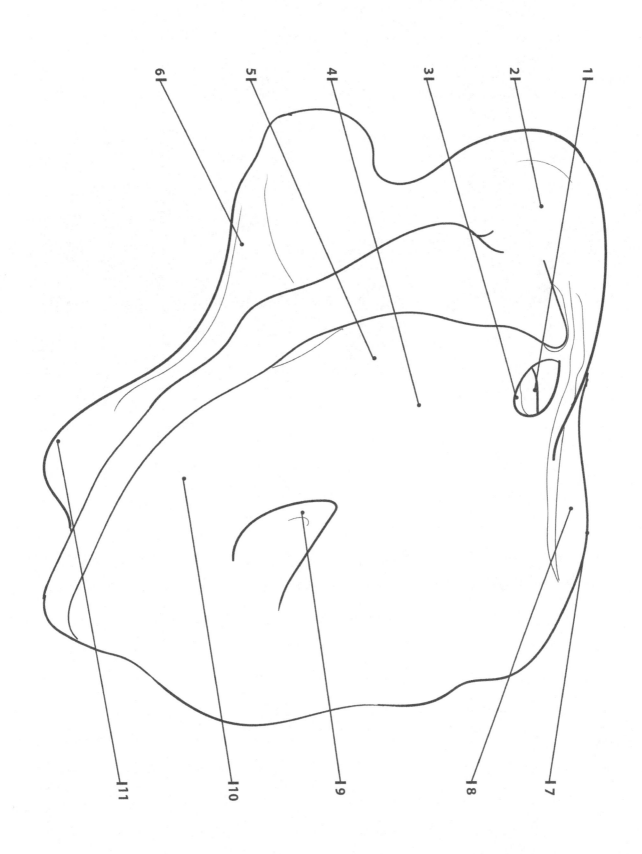

Horse - Atlas - C1 (Lateral view)

1. Lateral venebral foramen
2. Atlas
3. Alar foramen
4. Lateral mass
5. C1
6. Ventral arch

7. Dorsal tubercle
8. Dorsal arch
9. Transverse foramen
10. Transverse process[Atlantal wing]
11. Ventral tubercle

Horse - Atlas - C1 (Cranial view)

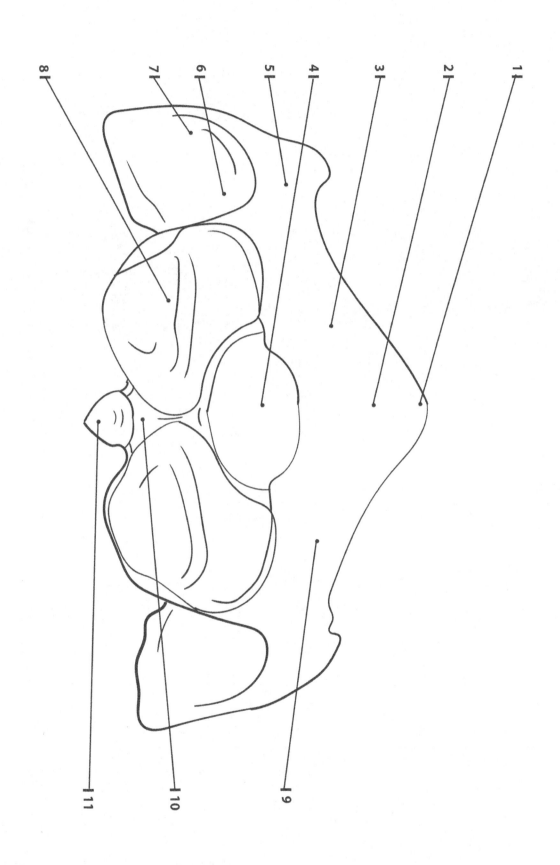

Horse - Atlas - C1 (Cranial view)

1. Dorsal tubercle
2. Dorsal arch
3. C1
4. Vertebral foramen
5. Lateral mass
6. Intraosseous canal
7. Transverse process[Atlantal wing]
8. Cranial articular fovea
9. Atlas
10. Ventral arch
11. Ventral tubercle

Horse - Atlas - C1 (Caudal view)

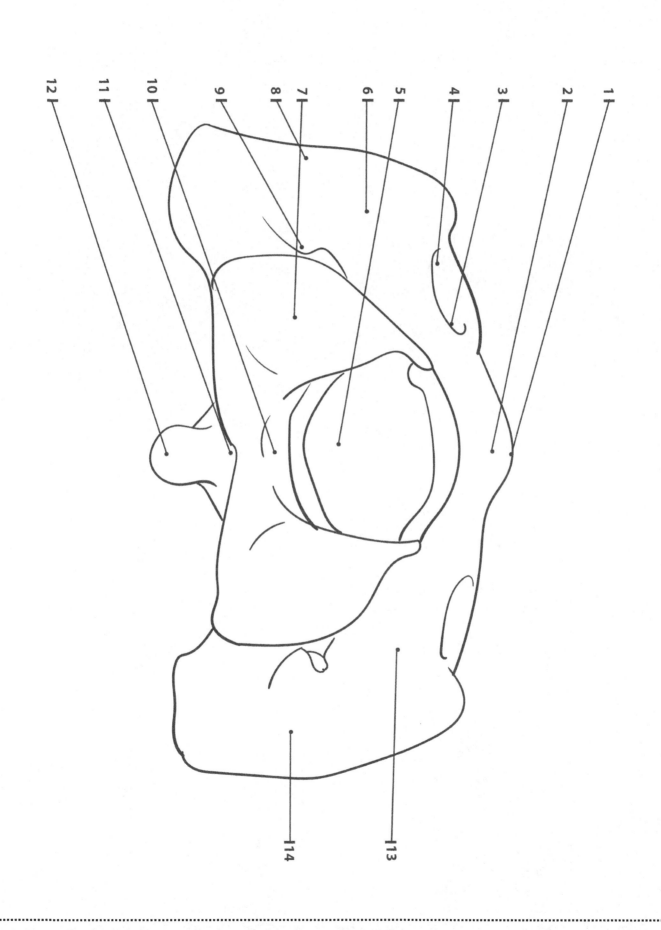

Horse - Atlas - C1 (Caudal view)

1. Dorsal tubercle
2. Dorsal arch
3. Lateral vertebral foramen
4. Alar foramen
5. Vertebral foramen
6. Lateral mass
7. Caudal articular fovea
8. Transverse process [Atlantal wing]
9. Transverse foramen
10. Fovea for dens
11. Ventral arch
12. Ventral tubercle
13. Atlas
14. C1

Horse - Atlas - C1 (Dorsal view)

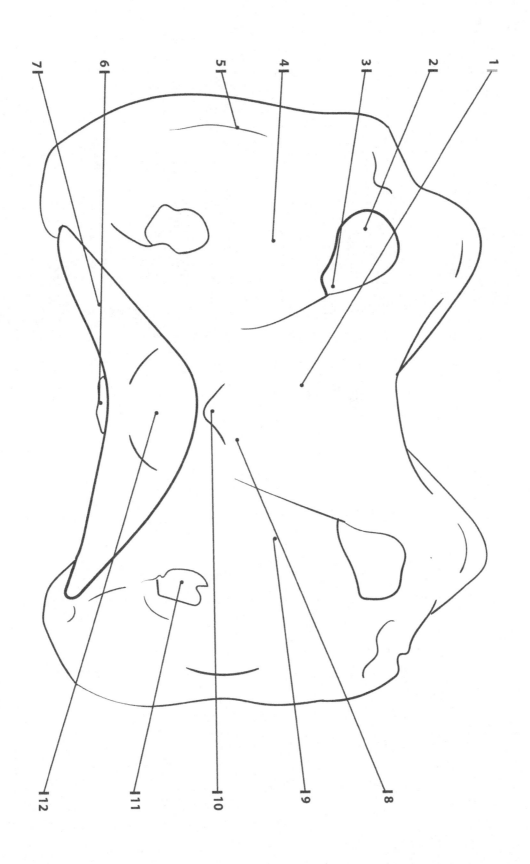

Horse - Atlas - C1 (Dorsal view)

1. Dorsal arch
2. Alar foramen
3. Lateral vertebral foramen
4. Lateral mass
5. Transverse process[Atlantal wing]
6. Ventral tubercle
7. Caudal articular fovea
8. C1
9. Atlas
10. Dorsal tubercle
11. Transverse foramen
12. Fovea for dens

Horse - Atlas- C1 (Ventral view)

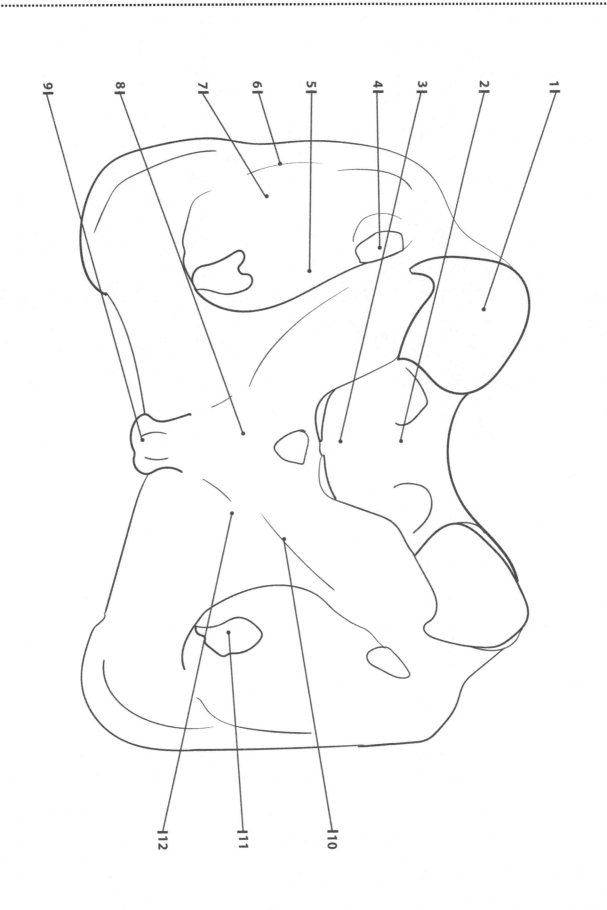

Horse - Atlas- C1 (Ventral view)

1.Cranial articular fovea
2.Dorsal arch
3.Vertebral foramen
4.Alar foramen
5.Lateral mass
6.Transverse process[Atlantal wing]
7.Intrasseous canal
8.Ventral arch
9.Ventral tubercle
10.Atlas
11.Transverse foramen
12.C1

Horse - Axis - C2 (Craniolateral view)

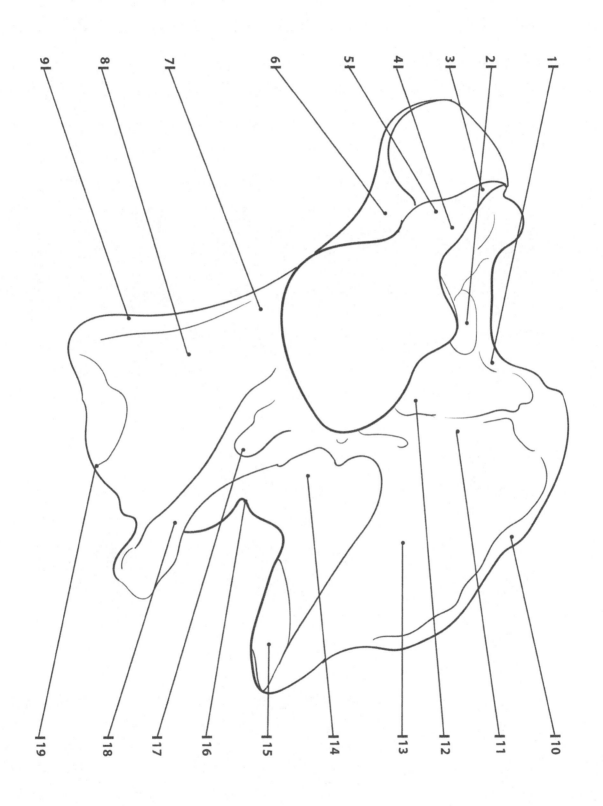

Horse - Axis - C2 (Craniolateral view)

1. Vertebral arch
2. Lateral vertebral foramen
3. Apex of the dens
4. Dens
5. Ventral articular facet of dens axis
6. Cranial extremity[Vertebral head]
7. C2
8. Vertebral body
9. Ventral crest
10. Spinous process
11. Lamina of vertebral arch
12. Vertebral foramen
13. Axis
14. Pedicle of vertebral arch
15. Caudal articular process
16. Caudal vertebral notch
17. Transverse foramen
18. Transverse process
19. Caudal extremity [Vertebral fossa]

Horse - Vertebra - C6 (Lateral view)

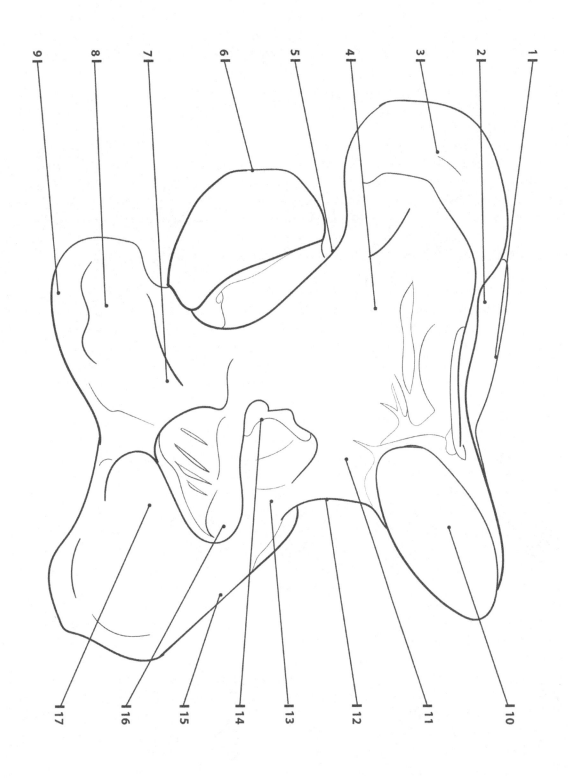

Horse - Vertebra - C6 (Lateral view)

1. Spinous process
2. Lamina of vertebral arch
3. Cranial articular process
4. Vertebral arch
5. Cranial vertebral notch
6. Cranial extremity[Vertebral head]
7. Transverse process
8. Ventral tubercle
9. Ventral plate
10. Caudal articular process
11. Pedicle of vertebral arch
12. Caudal vertebral notch
13. C6
14. Transverse foramen
15. Caudal extremity [Vertebral fossa]
16. Dorsal tubercle
17. Vertebral body

Horse - Vertebra - C6 (Cranial view)

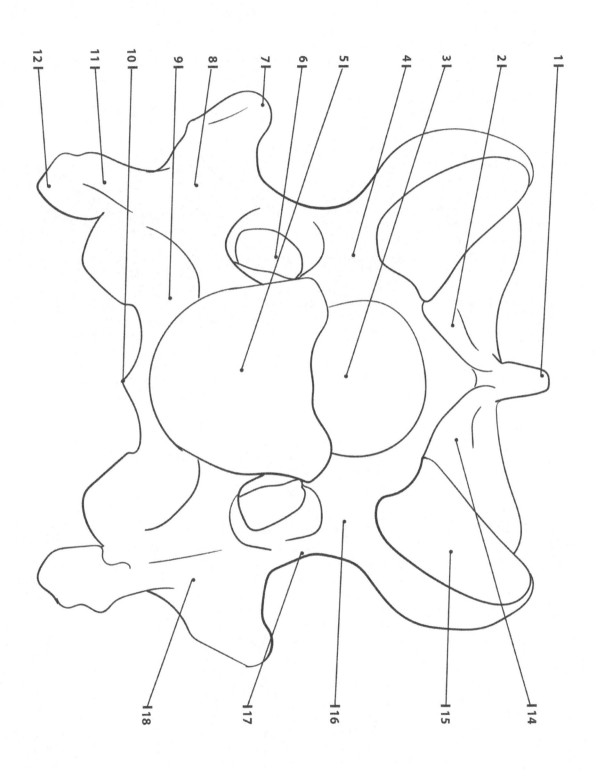

Horse - Vertebra - C6 (Cranial view)

1. Spinous process
2. Vertebral arch
3. Vertebral foramen
4. C6
5. Cranial extremity[Vertebral head]
6. Transverse foramen
7. Dorsal tubercle
8. Transverse process
9. Vertebral body
10. Ventral crest
11. Ventral tubercle
12. Ventral plate
13. Lamina of vertebral arch
14. Cranial articular process
15. Pedicle of vertebral arch
16. Cranial vertebral notch
17. Transverse process

Horse - Vertebra - C6 (Caudal view)

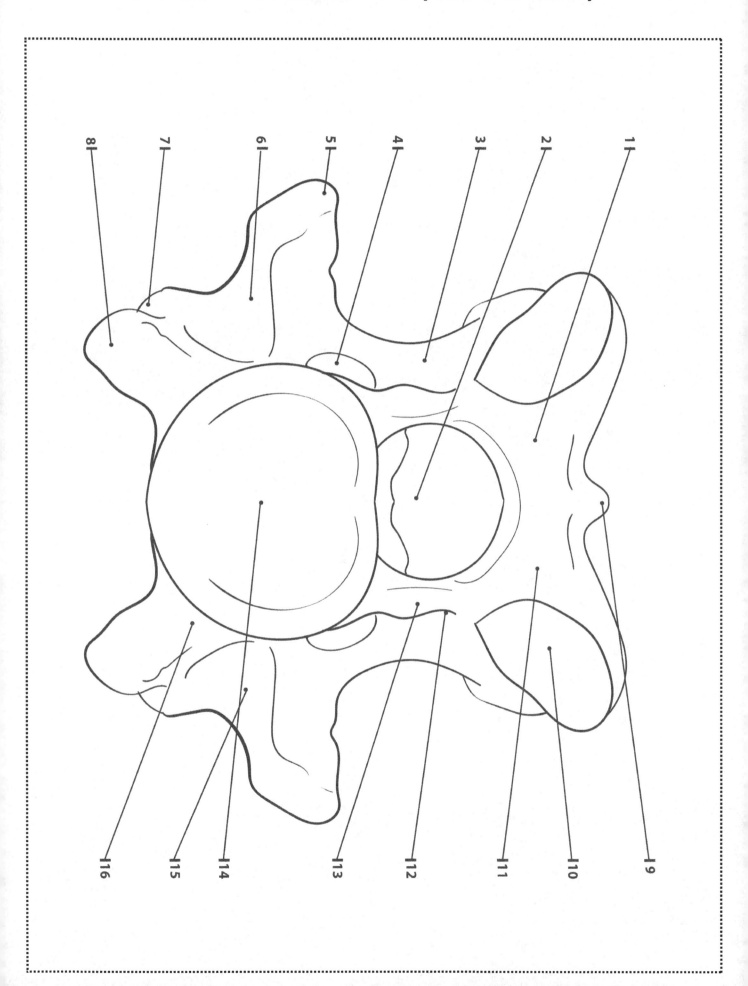

Horse - Vertebra - C6 (Caudal view)

1. Vertebral arch
2. Vertebral foramen
3. C6
4. Transverse foramen
5. Dorsal tubercle
6. Transverse process
7. Ventral plate
8. Ventral tubercle
9. Spinous process
10. Caudal articular process
11. Lamina of vertebral arch
12. Cadual vertebral notch
13. Pedicle of vertebral arch
14. Cadual extremity[Vertebral fossa]
15. Transverse process
16. Vertebral body

Horse - Vertebra - C6 (Dorsal view)

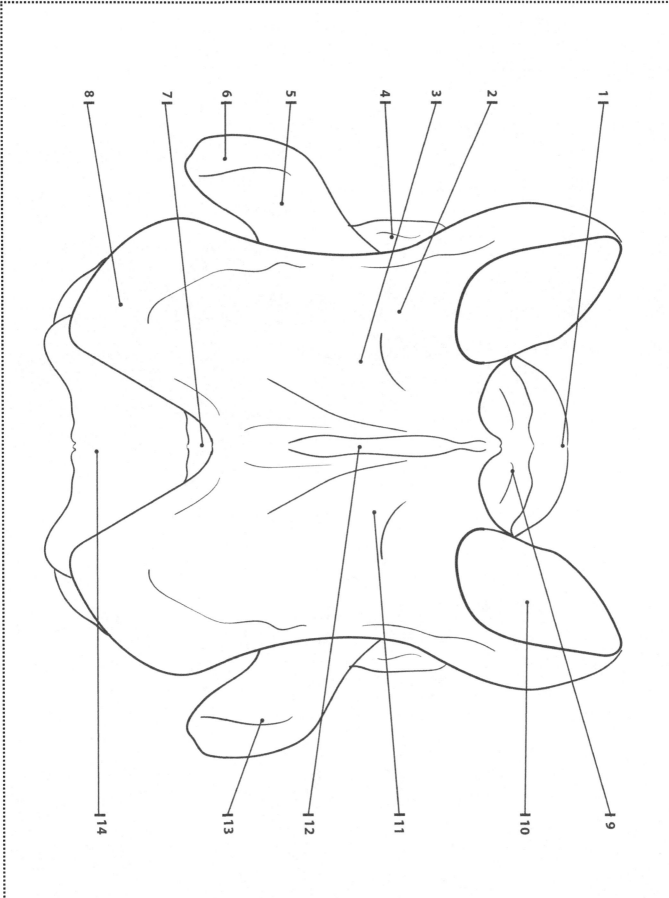

Horse - Vertebra - C6 (Dorsal view)

1. Carnial extremity [Vertebral head]
2. C6
3. Vertebral arch
4. Ventral plate
5. Transverse process
6. Dorsal tubercle
7. Vertebral foramen
8. Caudal articular process
9. Vertebral body
10. Carnial articular process
11. Lamina of vertebral arch
12. Spinous process
13. Transverse process
14. Cadual extremity[Vertebral fossa]

Horse - Vertebra - C6 (Ventral view)

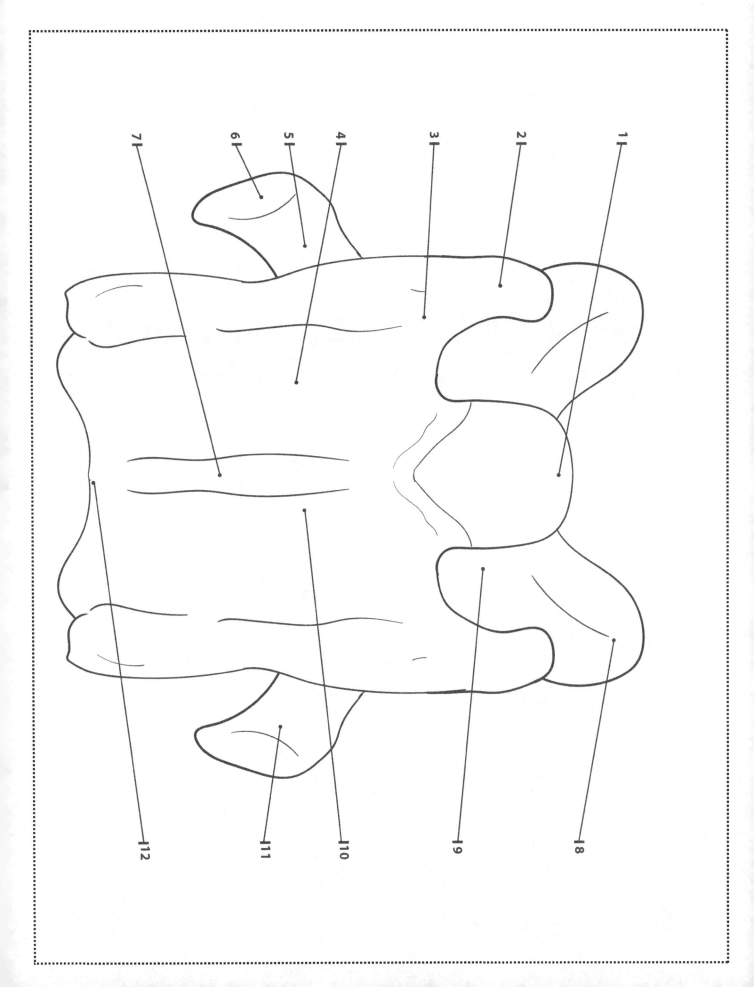

Horse - Vertebra - C6 (Ventral view)

1.Cranial extremity[Vertebral head]
2.Ventral plate
3.Ventral tubercle
4.C6
5.Transverse process
6.Dorsal tubercle
7.Ventral crest

8.Cranial articular process
9.Lamina of vertebral arch
10.Vertebral body
11.Transverse process
12.Caudal extremity[Vertebral fossa]

Horse - Thoracic vertebrae (Lateral view)

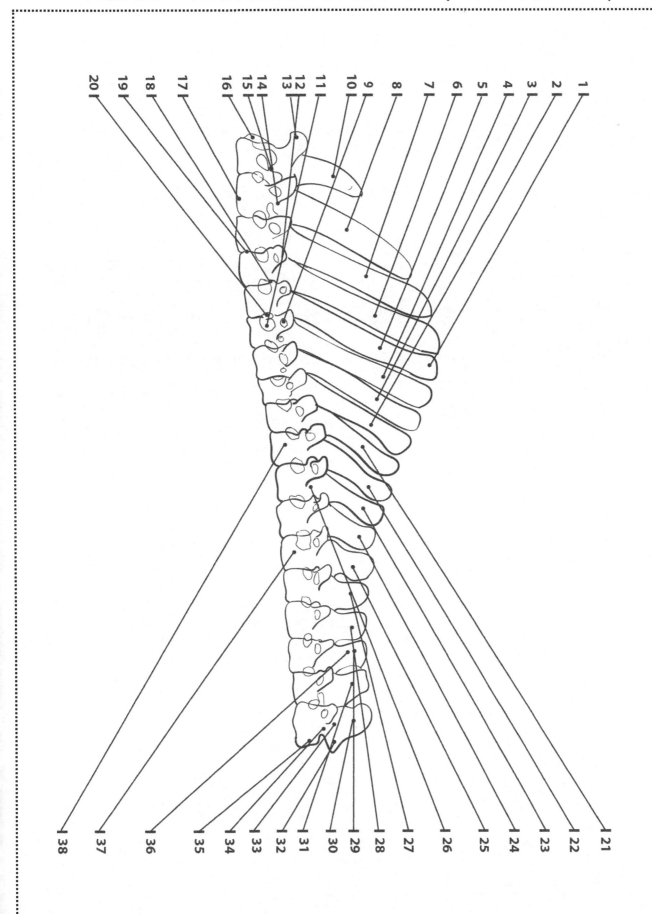

Horse - Thoracic vertebrae (Lateral view)

1. Spinous process
2. T8
3. T7
4. T6
5. T5
6. T4
7. T3
8. T2
9. Transverse costal facet
10. T1
11. Cranial costal facet
12. Transverse process
13. Cranial articular process
14. Vertebral arch
15. Intervertebral foramen
16. Cranial extremity [Vertebral head]
17. Ventral crest
18. Joints of articular processes
19. Intervertebral symphysis
20. Caudal costal facet
21. T9
22. T10
23. T11
24. T12
25. T13
26. Lateral vertebral foramen
27. T14
28. T15
29. Anticlinal vertebra
30. T18
31. T17
32. Caudal articular process
33. Lamina of vertebral arch
34. Pedicle of vertebral arch
35. Caudal extremity [Vertebral fossa]
36. T16
37. Vertebral body
38. Thoracic vertebrae

Horse - Thoracic vertebrae (Dorsal view)

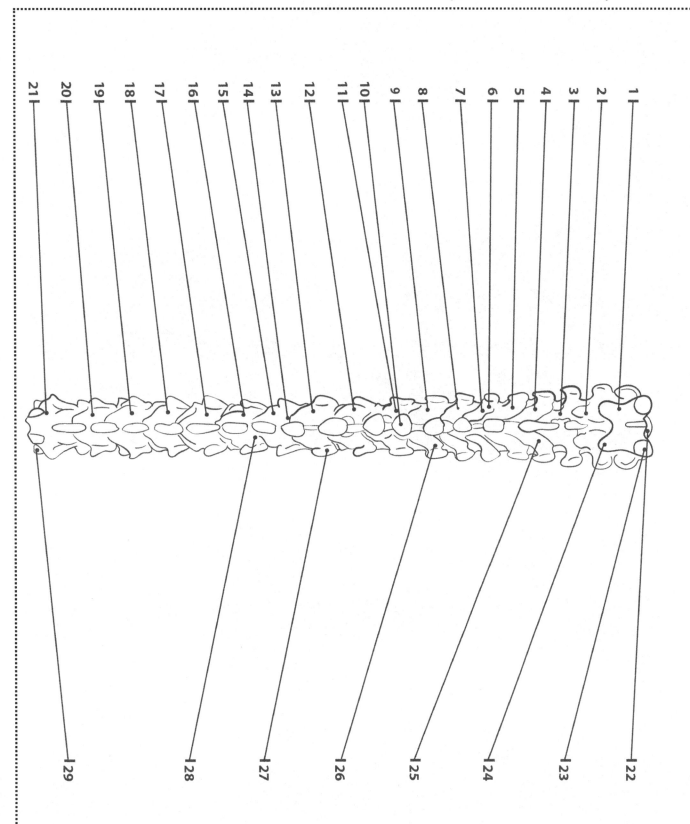

Horse - Thoracic vertebrae (Dorsal view)

1. T1
2. T2
3. T3
4. T4
5. T5
6. T6
7. Lamina of vertebral arch
8. T7
9. T8
10. Spinous process
11. T9
12. T10
13. T11
14. Interarcual space
15. T12
16. T13
17. T14
18. T15
19. T16
20. T17
21. T18

22. Cranial extremity [Vertebral head]
23. Cranial articular process
24. Caudal articular process
25. Vertebral arch
26. Thoracic vertebrae
27. Transverse process
28. Joints of articular processes
29. Caudal extremity [Vertebral fossa]

Horse - Vertebra-T6 (Lateral view)

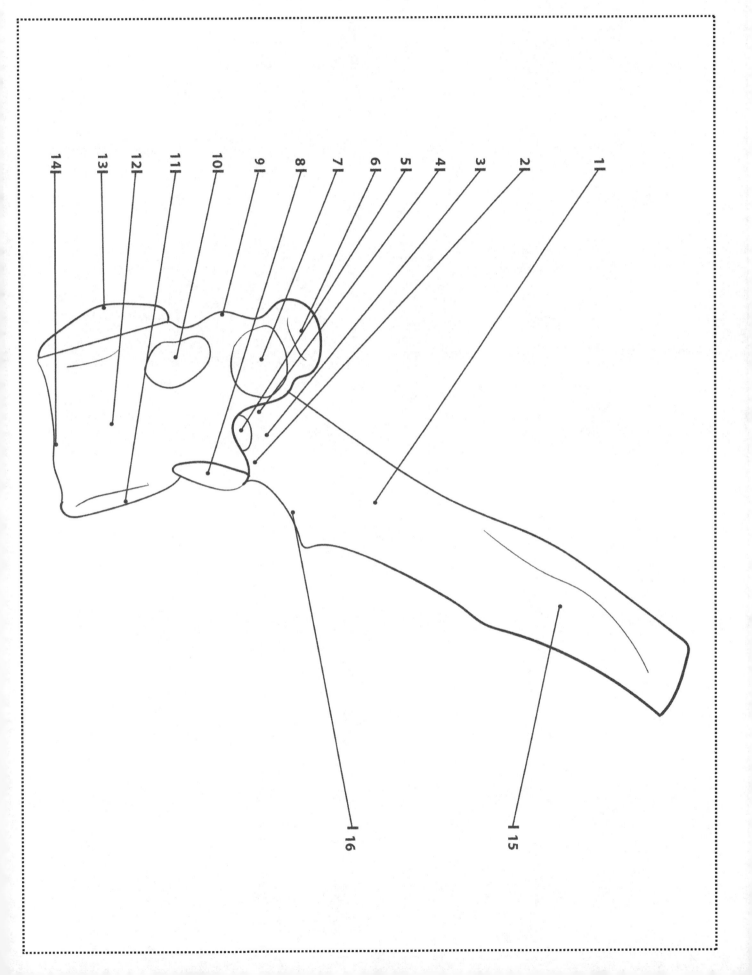

Horse - Vertebra-T6 (Lateral view)

1. T6
2. Pedicle of vertebral arch
3. Lamina of vertebral arch
4. Vertebral arch
5. Lateral vertebral foramen
6. Transverse process
7. Transverse costal facet
8. Caudal costal facet
9. Cranial articular process
10. Cranial costal facet
11. Caudal extremity [Vertebral fossa]
12. Vertebral body
13. Cranial extremity [Vertebral head]
14. Ventral crest
15. Spinous process
16. Caudal articular process

Horse - Vertebra - T6 (Cranial view)

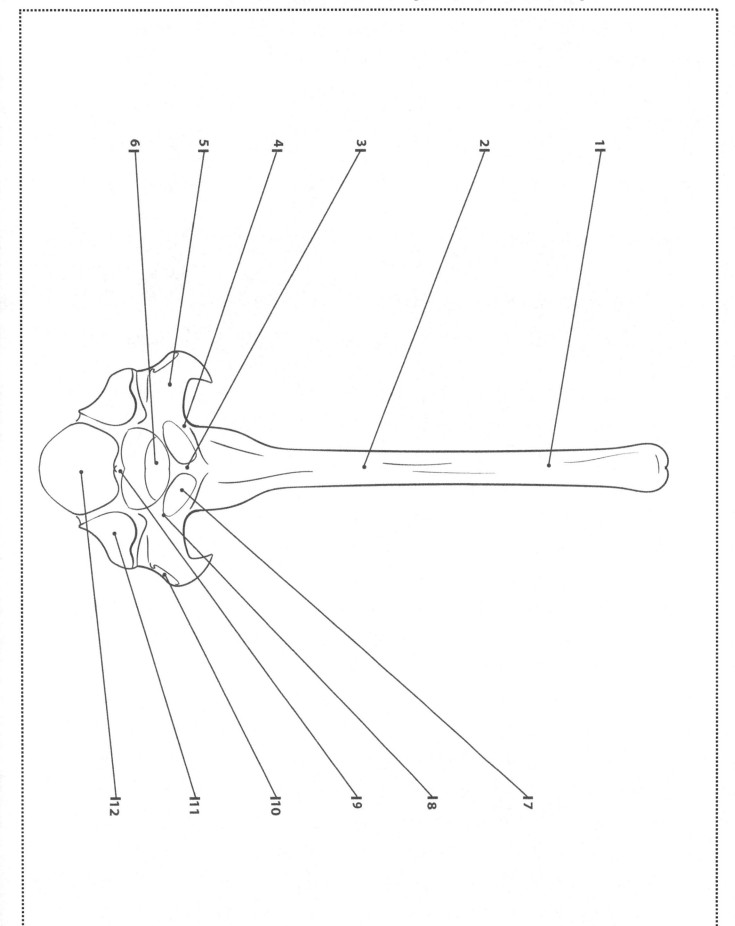

Horse - Vertebra - T6 (Cranial view)

1. Spinous process
2. T6
3. Lamina of vertebral arch
4. Vertebral arch
5. Transverse process
6. Vertebral foramen
7. Cranial articular process
8. Pedicle of vertebral arch
9. Vertebral body
10. Transverse costal facet
11. Cranial costal facet
12. Cranial extremity [Vertebral head]

Horse - Vertebra - T6 (Caudal view)

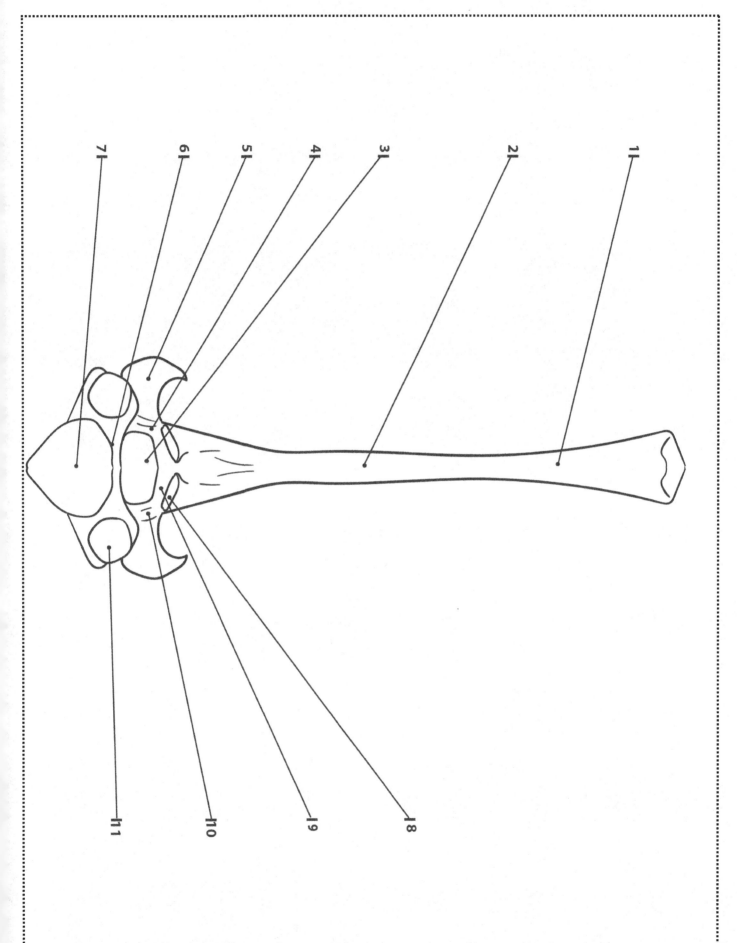

Horse - Vertebra - T6 (Caudal view)

1. Spinous process
2. T6
3. Vertebral foramen
4. Vertebral arch
5. Transverse process
6. Vertebral body
7. Caudal extremity [Vertebral fossa]
8. Caudal articular process
9. Lamina of vertebral arch
10. Pedicle of vertebral arch
11. Caudal costal facet

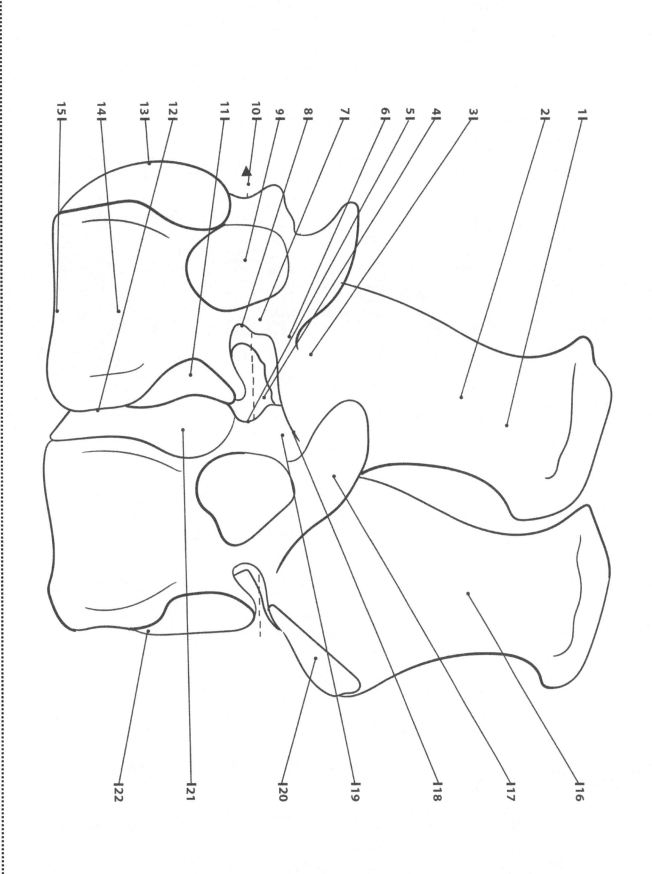

Horse - Vertebrae - T14/T15 (Lateral view)

1. Spinous process
2. T14
3. Lamina of vertebral arch
4. Intervertebral foramen
5. Cranial vertebral notch
6. Vertebral arch
7. Pedicle of vertebral arch
8. Caudal vertebral notch
9. Transverse costal facet
10. Vertebral canal
11. Caudal costal facet
12. Intervertebral symphysis
13. Cranial extremity [Vertebral head]
14. Vertebral body
15. Ventral crest
16. T15
17. Transverse process
18. Joints of articular processes
19. Cranial articular process
20. Caudal articular process
21. Cranial costal facet
22. Caudal extremity [Vertebral fossa]

Horse - Lumbar vertebrae (Lateral view)

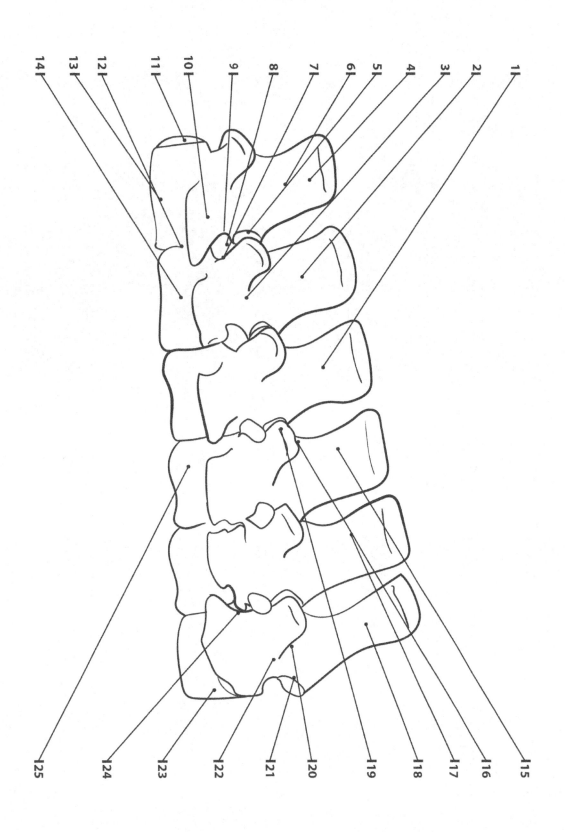

Horse - Lumbar vertebrae (Lateral view)

1. L3
2. L2
3. Vertebral arch
4. Spinous process
5. Joints of articular processes
6. L1
7. Cranial vertebral notch
8. Intervertebral foramen
9. Caudal vertebral notch
10. Costal process (Transverse proce
11. Cranial extremity [Vertebral head]
12. Intervertebral symphysis
13. Ventral crest
14. Lumbar vertebrae
15. L4
16. Mammillary process
17. L5
18. L6
19. Cranial articular process
20. Lamina of vertebral arch
21. Caudal articular process
22. Pedicle of vertebral arch
23. Caudal extremity [Vertebral fossa]
24. Lumbar intertransversar joi
25. Vertebral body

Horse - Lumbar vertebrae (Dorsal view)

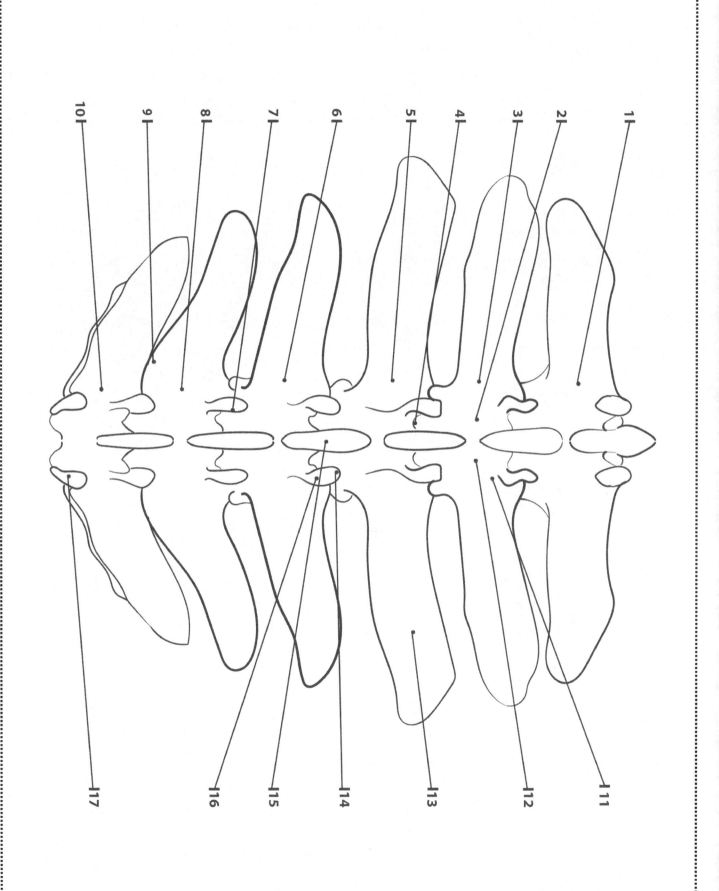

Horse - Lumbar vertebrae (Dorsal view)

1. L1
2. Vertebral arch
3. L2
4. Interarcual space
5. L3
6. L4
7. Joints of articular processes
8. L5
9. Lumbar intertransversar joint
10. L6
11. Pedicle of vertebral arch
12. Lamina of vertebral arch
13. Costal process [Transverse proces]
14. Cranial articular process
15. Spinous process
16. Mammillary process
17. Caudal articular process

Horse - Vertebra - L3 (Lateral view)

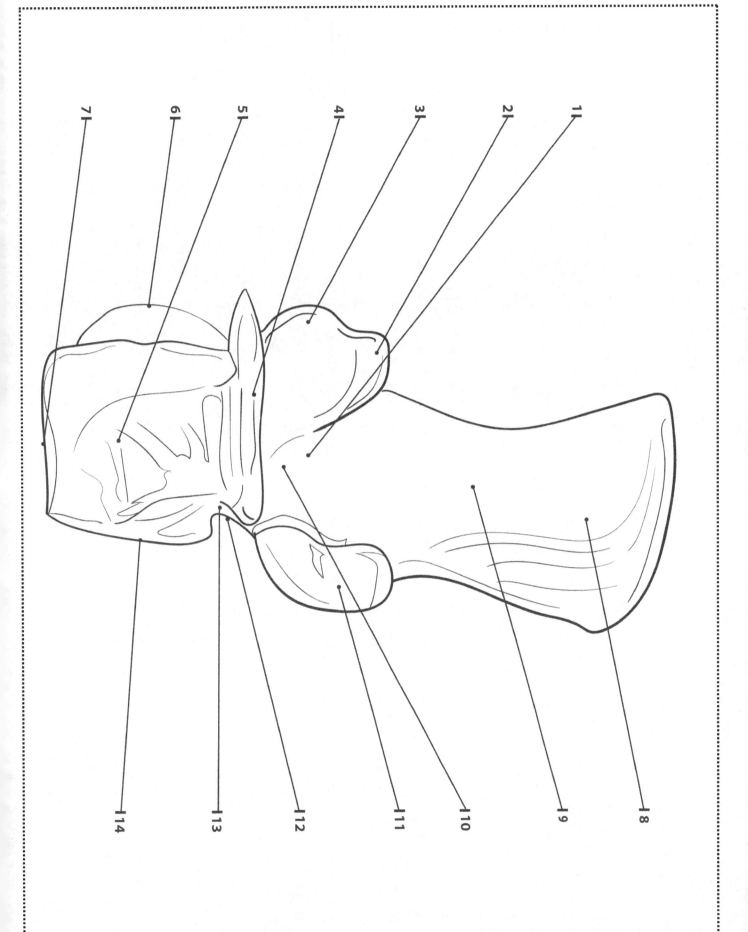

Horse - Vertebra - L3 (Lateral view)

1. Lamina of vertebral arch
2. Mammillary process
3. Cranial articular process
4. Costal process [Transverse process]
5. Vertebral body
6. Cranial extremity [Vertebral head]
7. Ventral crest
8. Spinous process
9. L3
10. Vertebral arch
11. Caudal articular process
12. Caudal vertebral notch
13. Pedicle of vertebral arch
14. Caudal extremity [Vertebral fossa]

Horse - Vertebra - L3 (Cranial view)

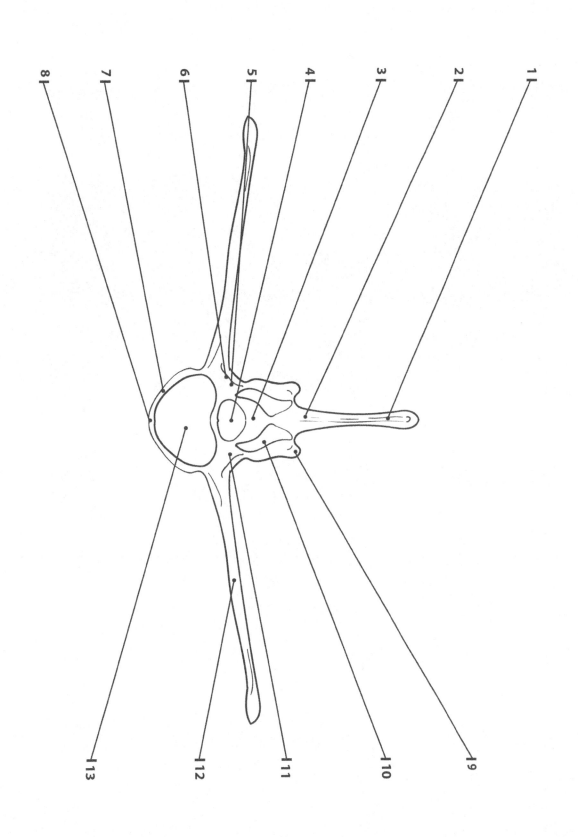

Horse - Vertebra - L3 (Cranial view)

1. Spinous process
2. L3
3. Lamina of vertebral arch
4. Vertebral foramen
5. Vertebral arch
6. Carnial vertebral notch
7. Vertebral body
8. Ventral crest
9. Mammillary process
10. Cranial articular process
11. Pedicle of vertebral arch
12. Costal process [Transverse process]
13. Cranial extremity [Vertebral head]

Horse - Vertebra - L3 (Caudal view)

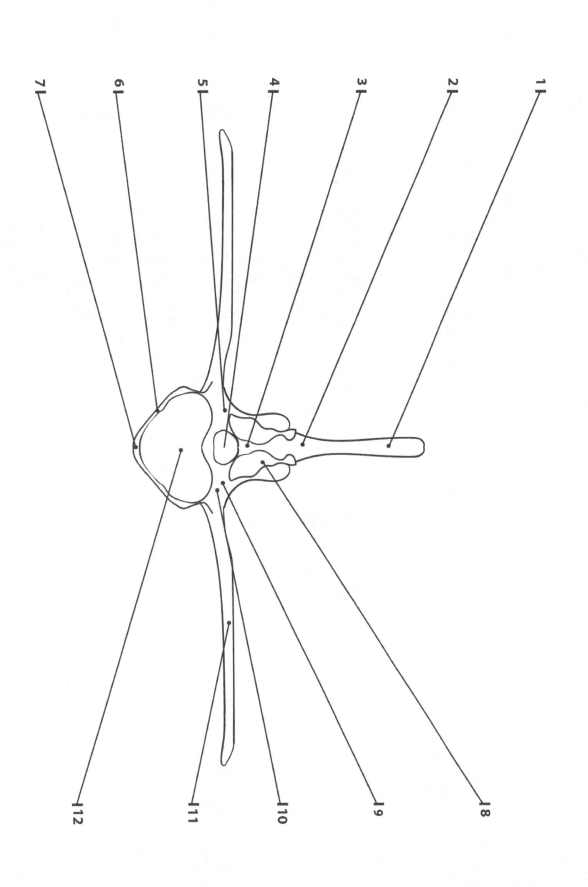

Horse - Vertebra - L3 (Caudal view)

1. Spinous process
2. L3
3. Lamina of vertebral arch
4. Vertebral foramen
5. Vertebral arch
6. Vertebral body
7. Ventral crest
8. Caudal articular process
9. Pedicle of vertebral arch
10. Caudal vertebral notch
11. Costal process [Transverse process]
12. Caudal extremity [Vertebral fossa]

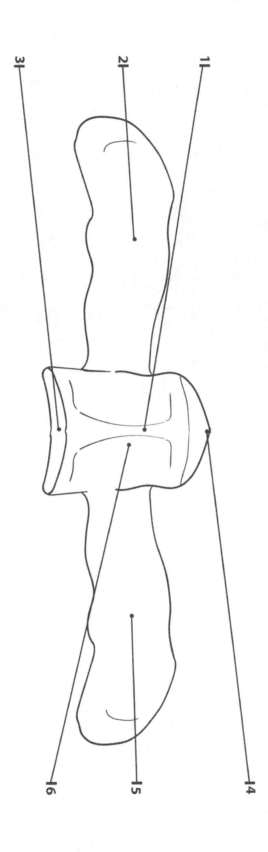

1.Ventral crest

2.L3

3.Caudal extremity[Vertebral fossa]

4.Cranial extremity [Vertebral head]

5.Costal process [Transverse process]

6.Vertebral body

Horse - Vertebrae - L3/L4 (Dorsal view)

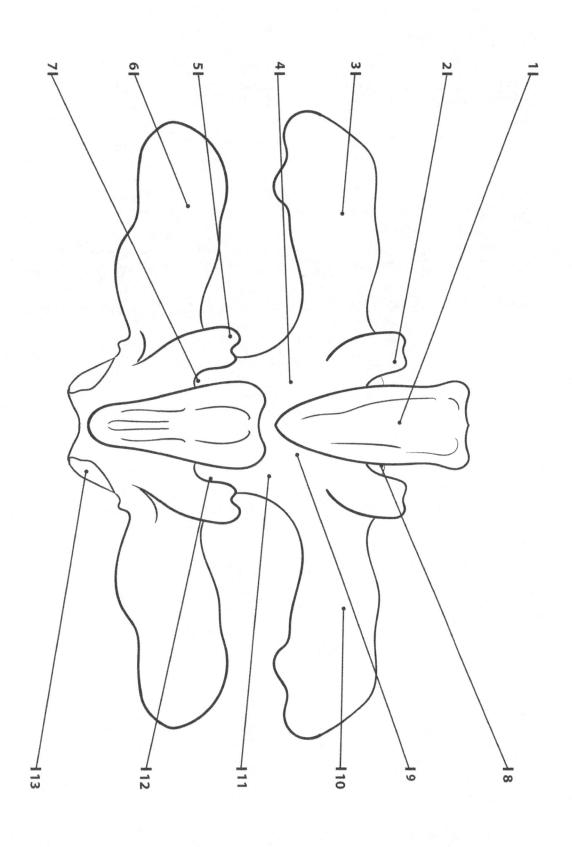

Horse - Vertebrae - L3/L4 (Dorsal view)

1. Spinous process
2. Cranial articular process
3. L3
4. Vertebral arch
5. Mammillary process
6. L4
7. Interarcual space
8. Cranial extremity[Vertebral head]
9. Lamina of vertebral arch
10. Costal process [Transverse proce]
11. Pedicle of vertebral arch
12. Joints of articular processes
13. Caudal articular process

Horse - Sacrum (Lateral view)

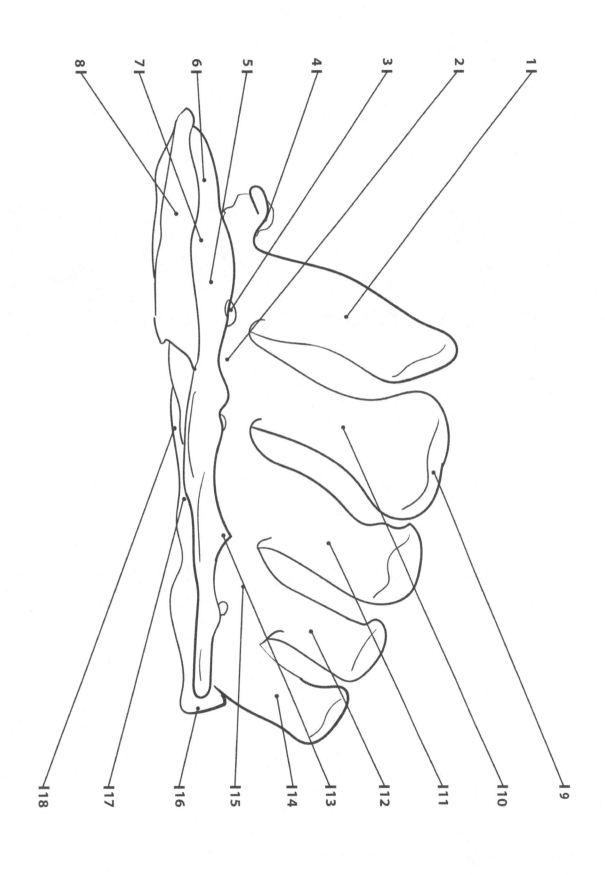

Horse - Sacrum (Lateral view)

1. S1
2. Dorsal surface
3. Dorsal sacral foramina
4. Cranial articular process
5. Sacral tuberosity
6. Ala(Wing of sacrum)
7. Lateral part of sacrum
8. Auricular surface
9. Median sacral crest
10. S2
11. S3
12. S4
13. Lateral sacral crest
14. S5
15. Sacrum [Sacral vertebrae]
16. Apex of sacrum
17. Ventral sacral foramina
18. Pelvic surface

Horse - Sacrum (Sagittal cross section)

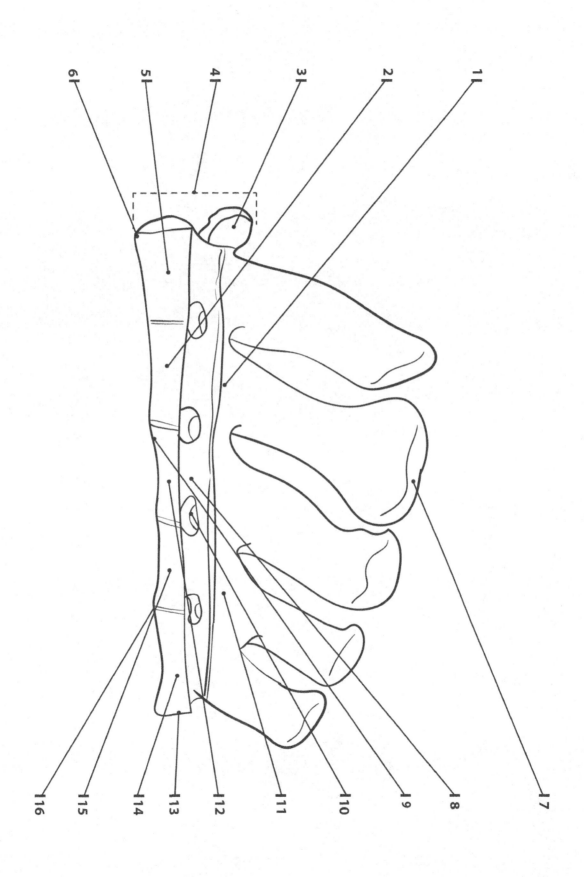

Horse - Sacrum (Sagittal cross section)

1. Dorsal surface
2. S2
3. Cranial articular process
4. Base of sacrum
5. S1
6. Promontory
7. Median sacral crest
8. Sacral canal
9. Pelvic surface
10. Intervertebral foramina
11. Sacrum [Sacral vertebrae]
12. S3
13. Apex of sacrum
14. S5
15. S4
16. Transverse lines

Horse - Sacrum (Cranial view)

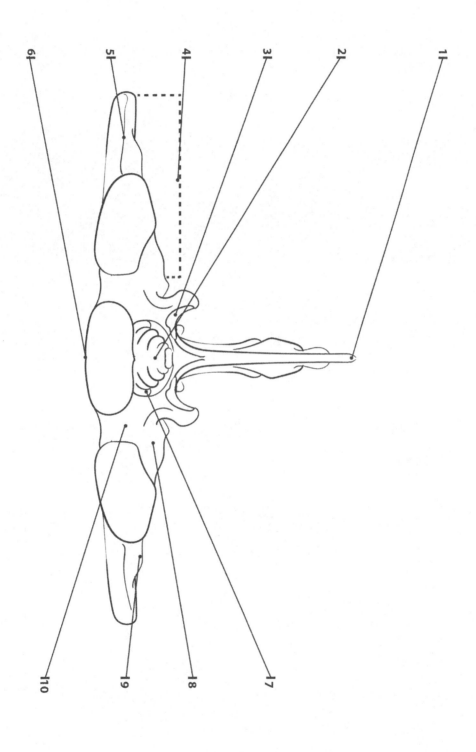

Horse - Sacrum (Cranial view)

1. Median sacral crest
2. Sacral canal
3. Cranial articular process
4. Lateral part of sacrum
5. Ala(Wing of sacrum)
6. Promontory
7. Intervertebral foramina
8. Dorsal surface
9. Sacral tuberosity
10. Sacrum [Sacral vertebrae]

Horse - Sacrum (Caudal view)

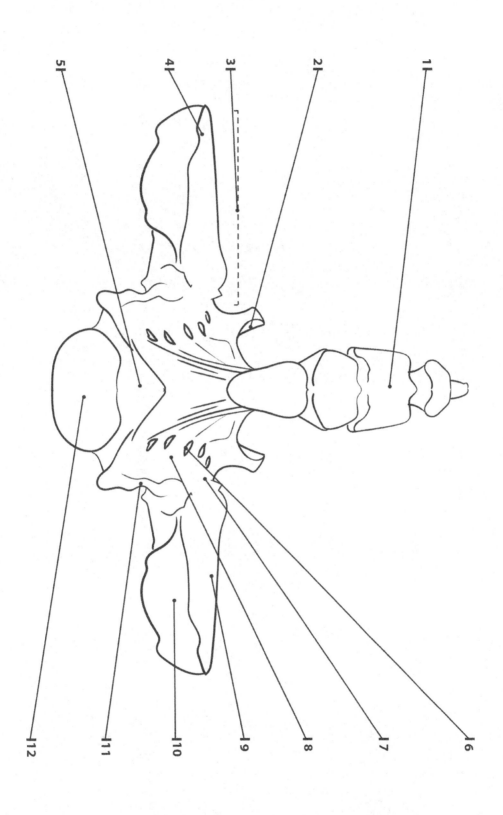

Horse - Sacrum (Caudal view)

1.Median sacral crest
2.Cranial articular process
3.Lateral part of sacrum
4.Ala; Wing of sacrum
5.Sacral canal

6.Dorsal sacral foramina
7.Sacrum [Sacral vertebrae]
8.Dorsal surface
9.Sacral tuberosity
10.Auricular surface
11.Lateral sacral crest
12.Apex of sacrum

Horse - Sacrum (Dorsal view)

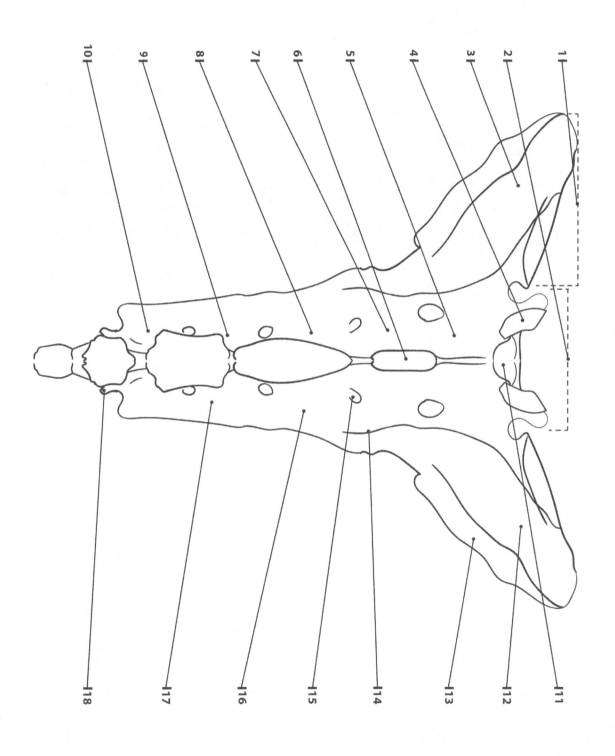

Horse - Sacrum (Dorsal view)

1. Lateral part of sacrum
2. Base of sacrum
3. Ala: Wing of sacrum
4. Cranial articular process
5. S1
6. Median sacral crest
7. S2
8. S3
9. S4
10. S5
11. Sacral canal
12. Sacral tuberosity
13. Auricular surface
14. Lateral sacral crest
15. Dorsal sacral foramina
16. Dorsal surface
17. Sacrum [Sacral vertebrae]
Apex of sacrum

Horse - Sacrum (Ventral view)

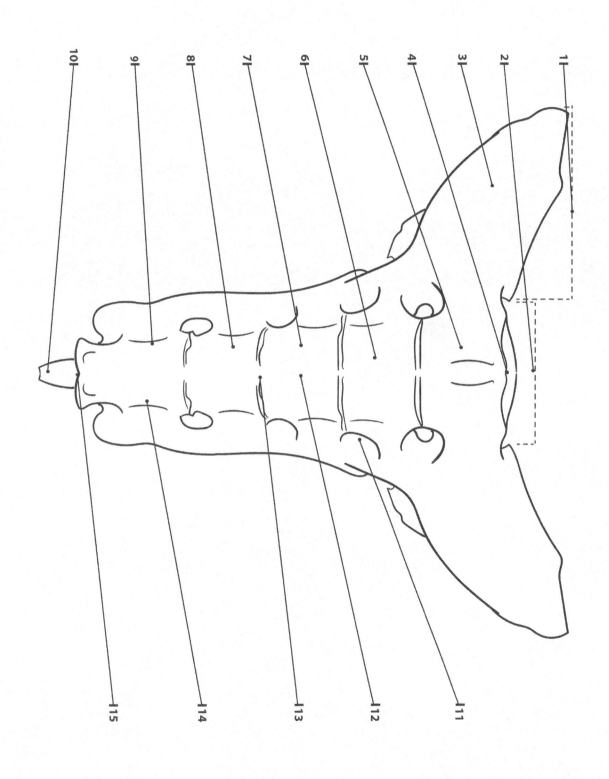

Horse - Sacrum (Ventral view)

1. Lateral part of sacrum
2. Base of sacrum
3. Ala : Wing of sacrum
4. Promontory
5. S1
6. S2
7. S3
8. S4
9. S5
10. Median sacral crest
11. Ventral sacral foramina
12. Pelvic surface
13. Transverse lines
14. Sacrum [Sacral vertebrae]
15. Apex of sacrum

Horse - Caudal vertebrae [Coccygeal] (Lateral view)

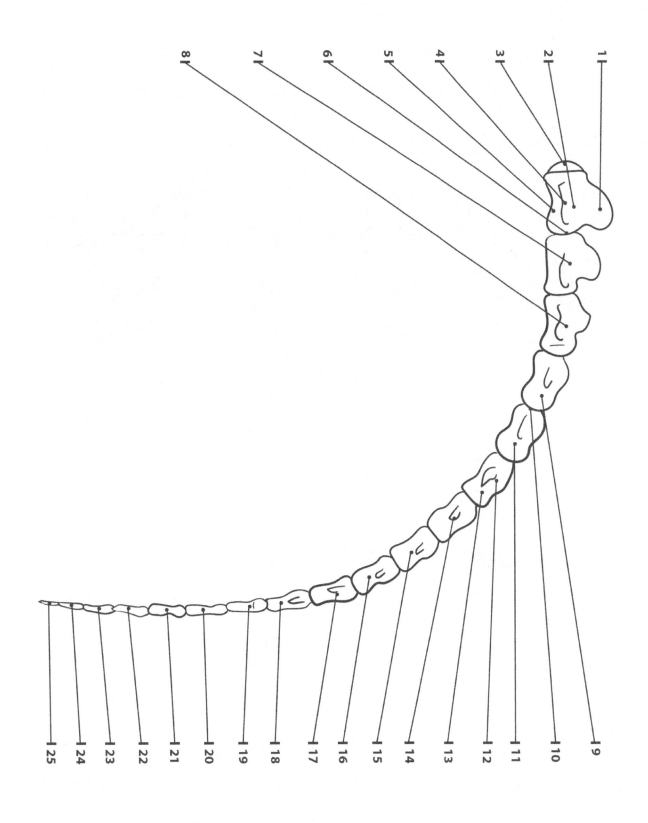

Horse - Caudal vertebrae [Coccygeal] (Lateral view)

1. Spinous process
2. Cd 1
3. Cranial extremity [Vertebral head]
4. Transverse process
5. Vertebral body
6. Caudal extremity [Vertebral fossa]
7. Cd 2
8. Cd 3
9. Cd 4
10. Intervertebral symphysis
11. Cd 5
12. Cd 6
13. Caudal vertebrae [Coccygeal]
14. Cd 7
15. Cd 8
16. Cd 9
17. Cd 10
18. Cd 11
19. Cd 12
20. Cd 13
21. Cd 14
22. Cd 15
23. Cd 16
24. Cd 17
25. Cd 18

Horse - Caudal vertebrae [Coccygeal] (Dorsal view)

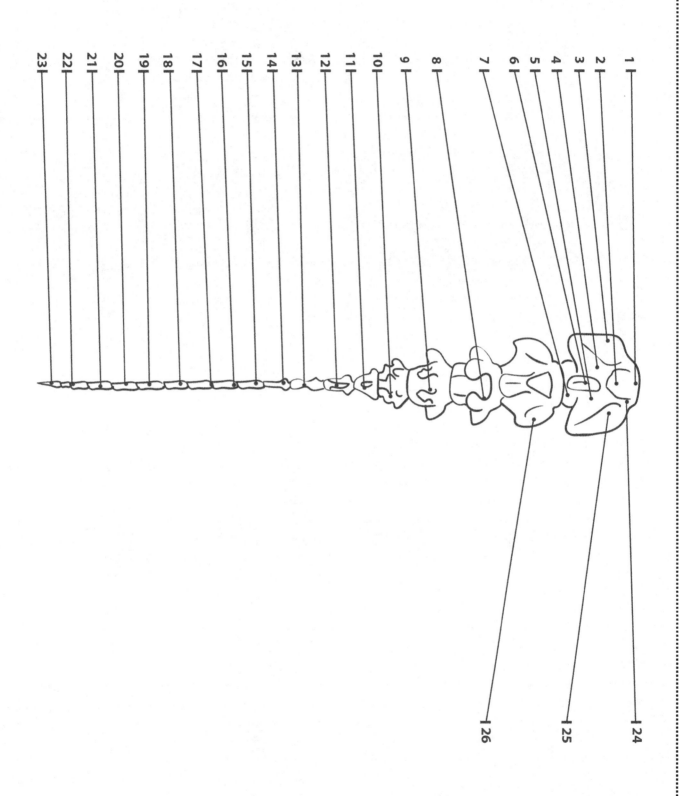

Horse - Caudal vertebrae [Coccygeal] (Dorsal view)

1.Cranial extremity [Vertebral head]
2.Vertebral foramen
3.Transverse process
4.Vertebral arch
5.Lamina of vertebral arch
6.Spinous process
7.Caudal extremity [Vertebral fossa]
8.Cd 3
9.Cd 4
10.Cd 5
11.Cd 6
12.Cd 7
13.Cd 8
14.Cd 9
15.Cd 10
16.Cd 11
17.Cd 12
18.Cd 13
19.Cd 14
20.Cd 15
21.Cd 16
22.Cd 17
23.Cd 18

24. Pedicle of vertebral arch
25. Cd 1
26. Cd 2

Horse - Vertebra - Cd 2 (Caudal view)

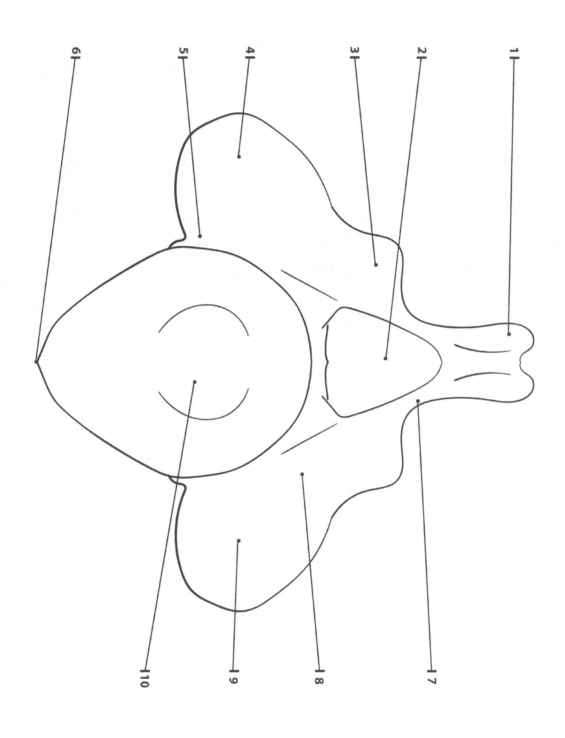

1. Spinous process
2. Vertebral foramen
3. Vertebral arch
4. Transverse process
5. Vertebral body
6. Ventral crest

7. Lamina of vertebral arch
8. Pedicle of vertebral arch
9. Cd 2
10. Caudal extremity [Vertebral fossa]

Horse - Thoracic skeleton (Lateral view)

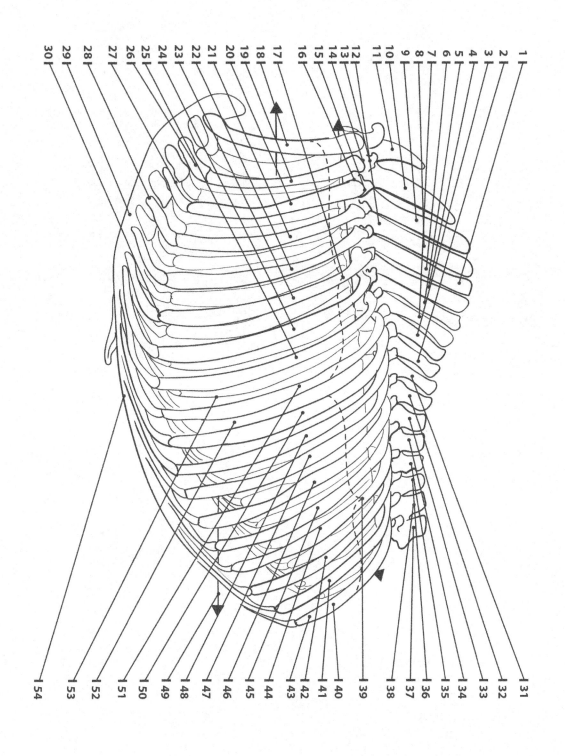

Horse - Thoracic skeleton (Lateral view)

1. Spinous process
2. T10
3. T9
4. T6
5. T7
6. T5
7. T8
8. T4
9. T3
10. T2
11. T1
12. Thoracic vertebrae
13. Transverse process
14. Costovertebral joints
15. Costotransverse joint
16. Joint of head of rib
17. True ribs [Sternal ribs]
18. Rib-1
19. Rib-2
20. Rib-3
21. Rib-4
22. Rib-5
23. Rib-6
24. Rib-7
25. Rib-8
26. Costal cartilage
27. Sternal synchondroses
28. Sternocostal joints
29. Sternum
30. Costochondral joints
31. T11
32. T12
33. T13
34. T14
35. T15
36. T16
37. T18
38. T17
39. False ribs [Asternal ribs]
40. Rib - 18
41. Rib - 17
42. Rib - 16
43. Floating ribs
44. Rib - 15
45. Rib - 14
46. Rib - 13
47. Rib - 12
48. Rib - 11
49. Caudal thoracic aperture
50. Rib - 10
51. Rib - 9
52. Intercostal space
53. Thoracic cavity
54. Costal arch

Horse - Thoracic skeleton (Dorsal view)

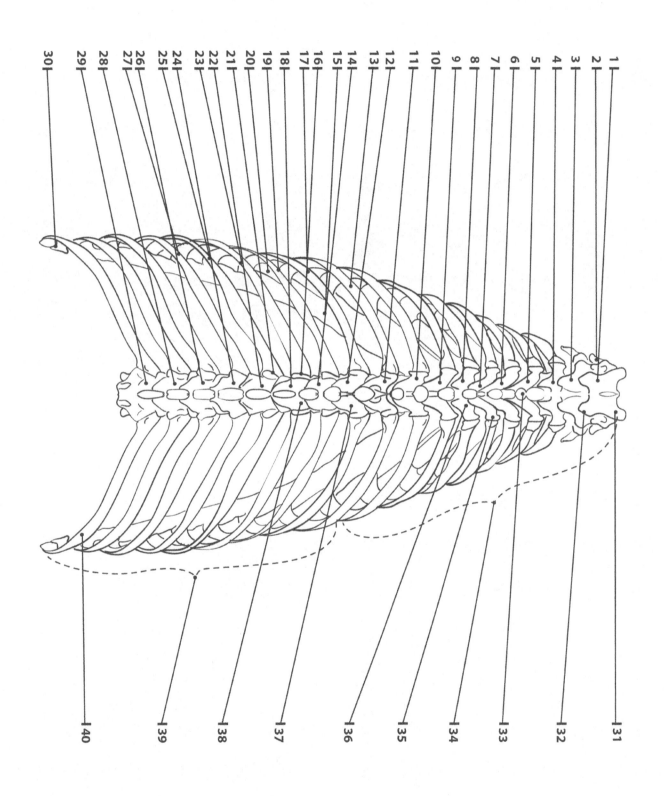

Horse - Thoracic skeleton (Dorsal view)

1. T1H
2. Rib-1
3. T2
4. T3
5. T4
6. T5
7. T6
8. T7
9. T8
10. T9
11. T10
12. T11
13. Rib-10
14. T12
15. Costal cartilage
16. Costovertebral joints
17. Rib-11
18. T13
19. Rib- 12
20. Thoracic cavity
21. Costotransverse joint
22. T14
23. Rib-13
24. T15
25. Rib- 14
26. T16
27. Rib- 15
28. T17
29. T18
30. Costochondral joints
31. Cranial articular process
32. Caudal articular process
33. Spinous process
34. True ribs [Sternal ribs]
35. Transverse process
36. Lamina of vertebral arch
37. Thoracic vertebrae
38. Joints of articular processes
39. False ribs [Asternal ribs]
40. Floating ribs

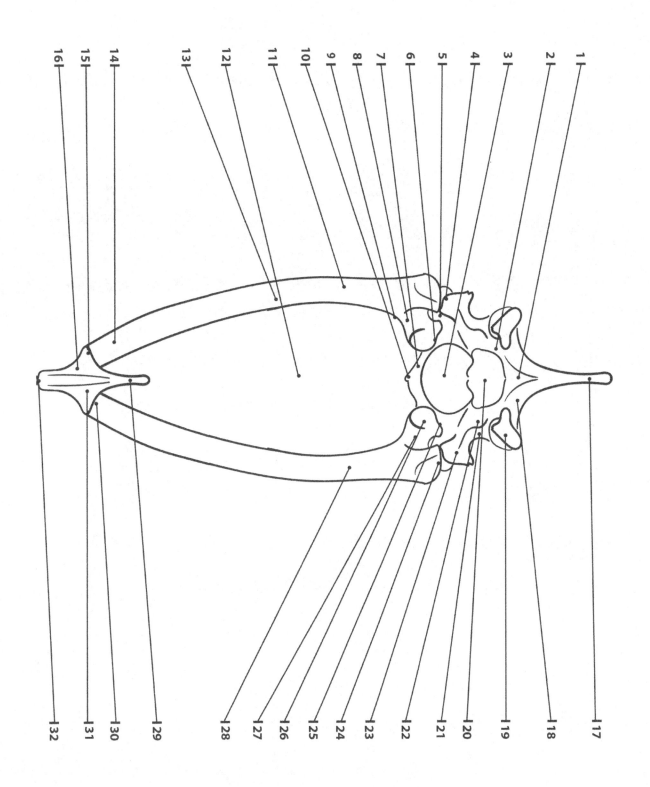

Horse - Cranial thoracic aperture (Cranial view)

1. T1
2. Vertebral arch
3. Cranial extremity [Vertebral head]
4. Costotransverse joint
5. Costotransverse foramen
6. Joint of head of rib
7. Vertebral body
8. Crest of costal neck
9. Costal angle
10. Ventral crest
11. Rib 1H
12. Cranial thoracic aperture
13. Ventral scalene muscle tubercle
14. Rib
15. Costal cartilage
16. Sternum
17. Spinous process
18. Lamina of vertebral arch
19. Cranial articular process
20. Vertebral foramen
21. Cranial vertebral notch
22. Pedicle of vertebral arch
23. Transverse process
24. Costal tubercle
25. Costovertebral joints
26. Costal head
27. Costal neck
28. Costal body [Shaft]
29. Cartilage of manubrium
30. Sternocostal joints
31. Manubrium of sternum
32. Sternal crest

Horse - Rib - 8 (Left) (Craniolateral view)

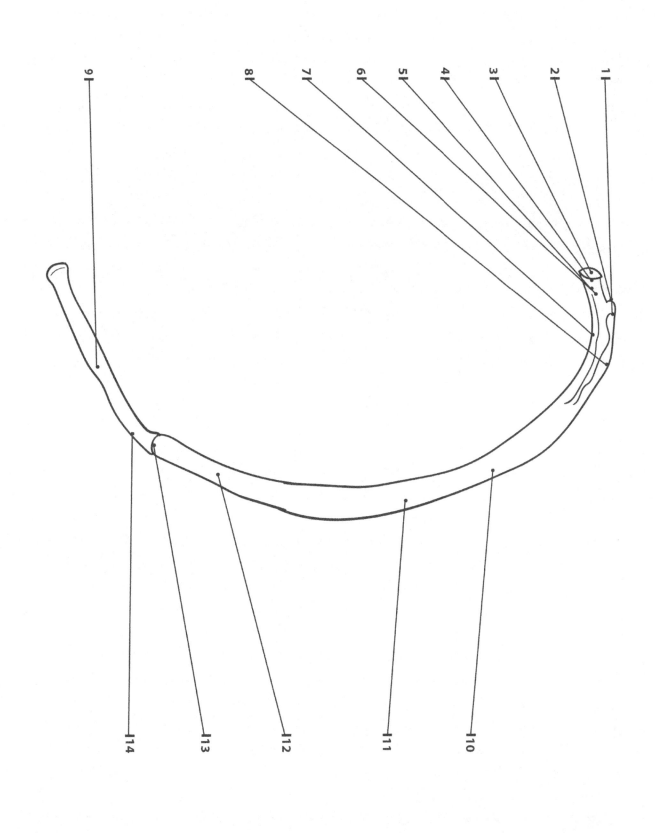

Horse - Rib - 8 (Left) (Craniolateral view)

1. Costal tubercle
2. Articular facet of costal tubercle
3. Articular facet of costal head
4. Costal head
5. Costal neck
6. Crest of costal neck
7. Costal angle
8. Longissimus muscle tubercle
9. Costal cartilage
10. Rib - 8
11. Costal body [Shaft]
12. Rib
13. Costochondral joints
14. Costal knee

Horse - Rib - 8 (Left) (Caudomedial view)

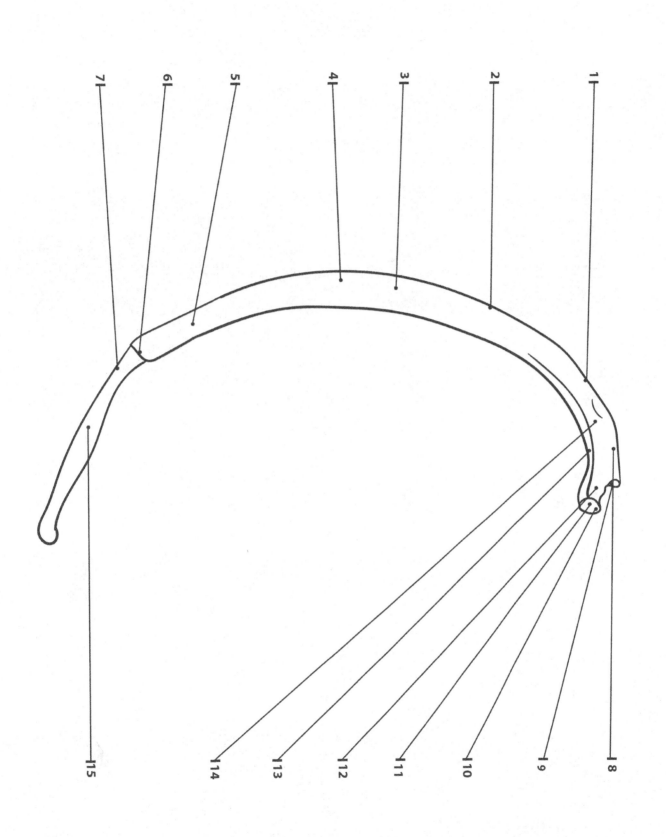

Horse - Rib - 8 (Left) (Caudomedial view)

1. Longissimus muscle tubercle
2. Iliocostal muscle tubercle
3. Costal body [Shaft]
4. Rib-8
5. Rib
6. Costochondral joints
7. Costal knee
8. Costal tubercle
9. Articular facet of costal tubercle
10. Articular facet of costal head
11. Costal head
12. Costal neck
13. Costal angle
14. Costal groove
15. Costal cartilage

Horse - Rib - 12 (Left) (Caudomedial view)

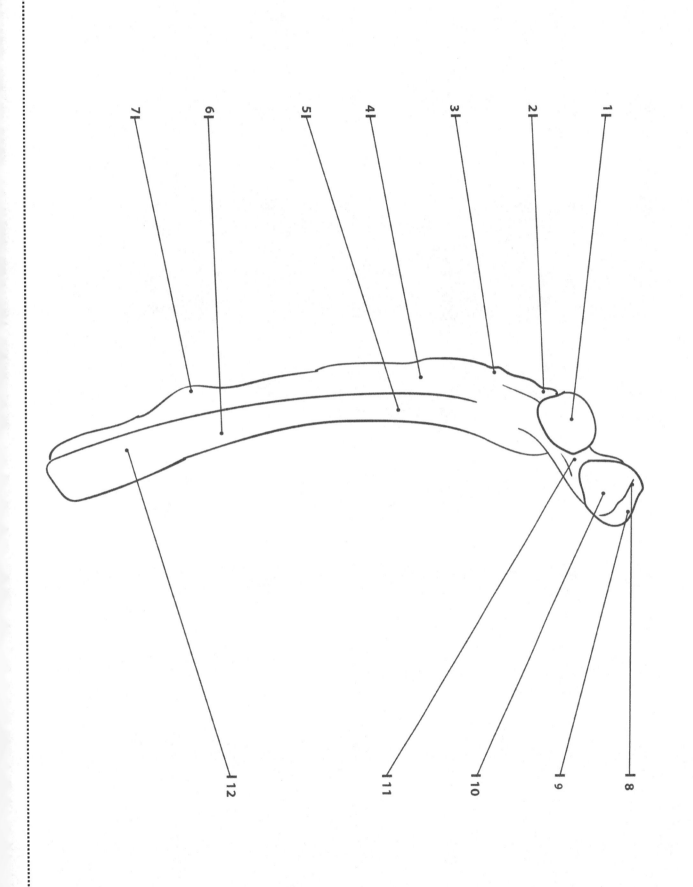

Horse - Rib - 12 (Left) (Caudomedial view)

1. Articular facet of costal tubercle
2. Costal tubercle
3. Longissimus muscle tubercle
4. Costal groove
5. Costal body [Shaft]
6. Rib
7. Iliocostal muscle tubercle

8. Costal head
9. Crest of costal head
10. Articular facet of costal head
11. Costal neck
12. Rib - 12

Horse -Sternum (Lateral view)

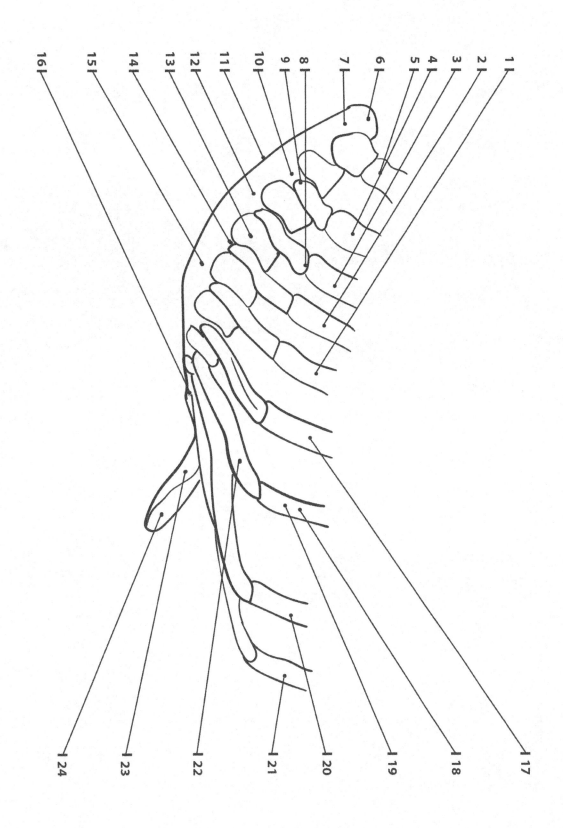

Horse -Sternum (Lateral view)

1. Rib-5
2. Rib-4
3. Rib 3
4. Rib-2
5. Rib 1
6. Cartilage of manubrium
7. Manubrium of sternum
8. Costochondral joints
9. Sternocostal joints
10. Manubriosternal synchondrosis
11. Sternal crest
12. Body of sternum
13. Sternebrae
14. Intersternebral synchondroses
15. Sternum
16. Xiphosternal synchondrose

17. Rib - 6
18. Rib - 7
19. Rib
20. Rib - 8
21. Rib - 9
22. Costal cartilage
23. Xiphoid process
24. Xiphoid cartilage

Horse - Sternum (Lateral view)

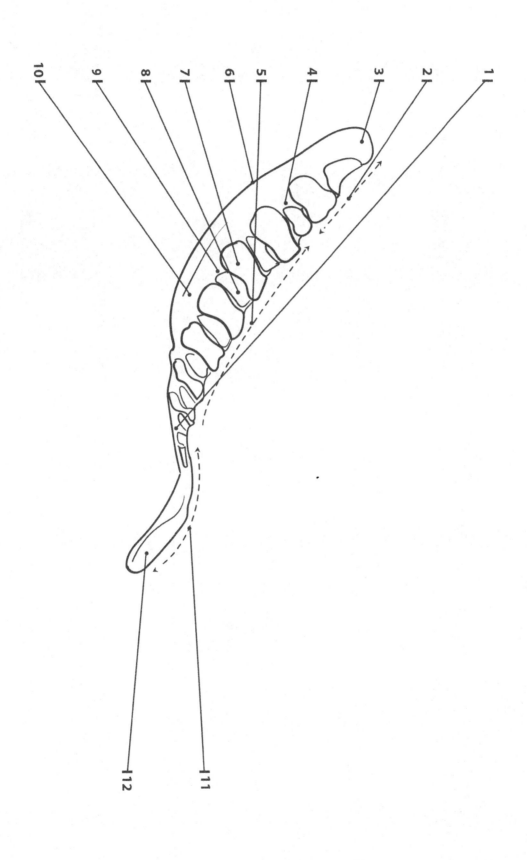

Horse - Sternum (Lateral view)

1. Xiphosternal synchondrose
2. Manubrium of sternum
3. Cartilage of manubrium
4. Manubriosternal synchondrosis
5. Body of sternum
6. Sternal crest
7. Sternebrae
8. Costal notches
9. Intersternebral synchondroses
10. Sternum
11. Xiphoid process
12. Xiphoid cartilage

Horse - Sternum (Dorsal view)

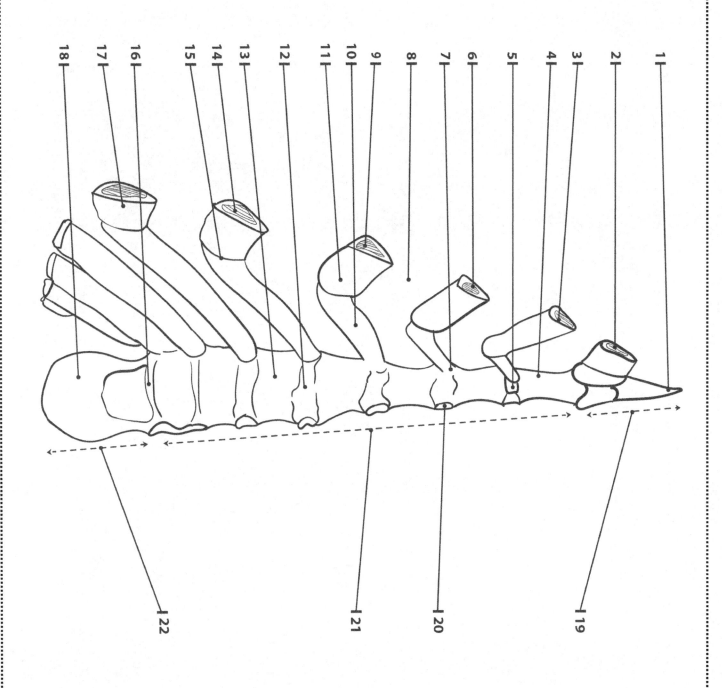

Horse - Sternum (Dorsal view)

1. Cartilage of manubrium
2. Rib 1
3. Rib 2
4. Sternum
5. Manubriosternal synchondrosis
6. Rib 3
7. Sternocostal joints
8. Intercostal space
9. Rib-4
10. Costal cartilage
11. Rib
12. Intersternebral synchondroses
13. Sternebrae
14. Rib 5
15. Costochondral joints
16. Xiphosternal synchondrosel
17. Rib 6
18. Xiphoid cartilage
19. Manubrium of sternum
20. Costal notches
21. Body of sternum
22. Xiphoid process

Horse -Sternum (Ventral view)

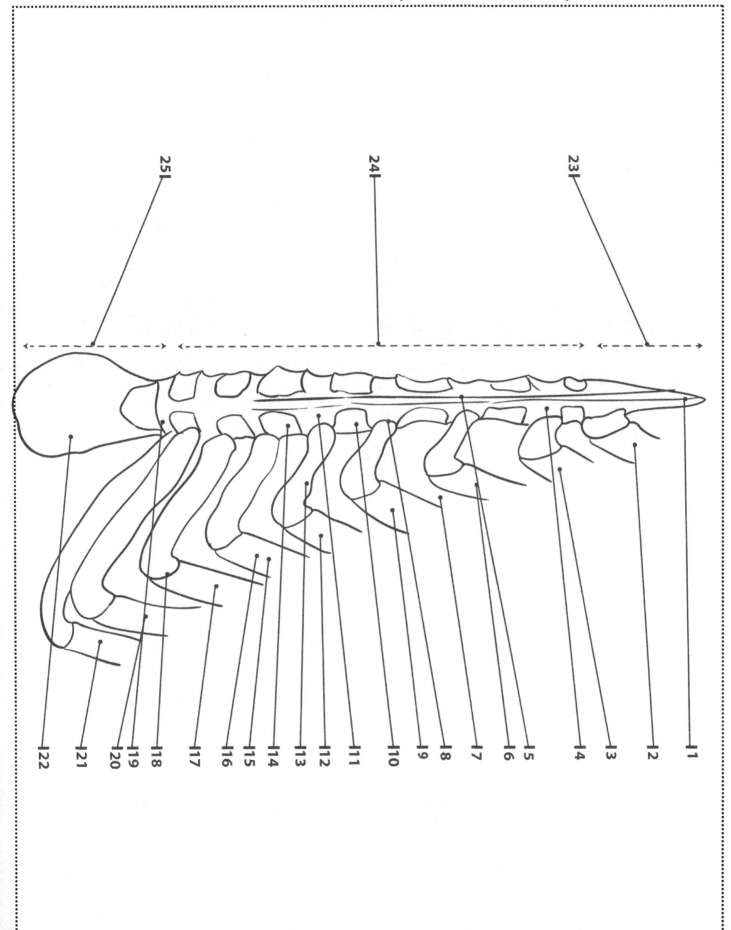

Horse -Sternum (Ventral view)

1. Cartilage of manubrium
2. Rib - 1
3. Rib-2
4. Manubriosternal synchondrosis
5. Sternal crest
6. Rib-3
7. Intercostal space
8. Sternocostal joints
9. Rib-4
10. Sternum
11. Intersternebral synchondroses
12. Rib
13. Costal cartilage
14. Sternebrae
15. Rib-6
16. Rib - 5
17. Rib - 7
18. Costochondral joints
19. Xiphosternal synchondrose
20. Rib - 8
21. Rib - 9
22. Xiphoid cartilage
23. Manubrium of sternum
24. Body of sternumH
25. Xiphoid process

Horse - Bones of the thoracic limb (Left) (Lateral view)

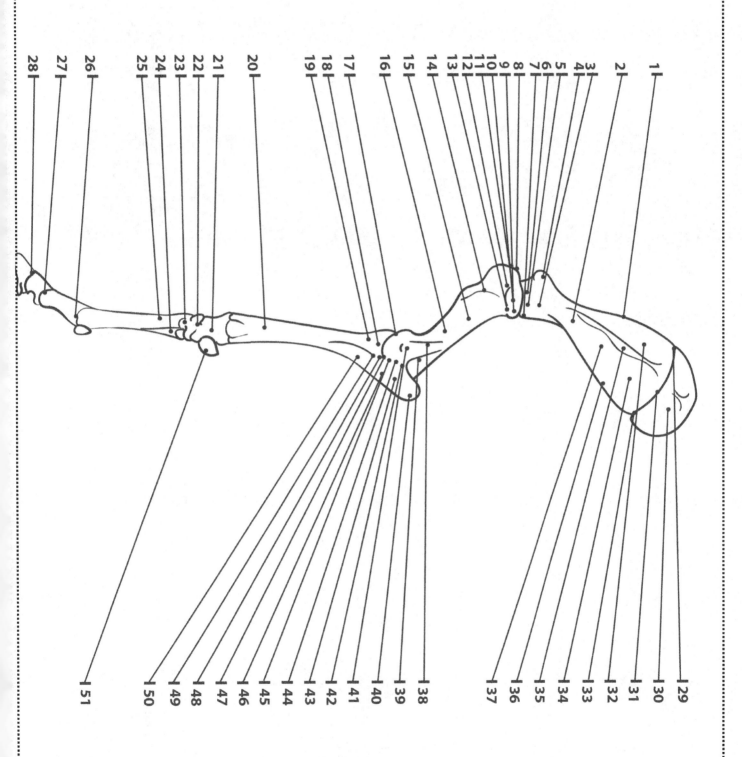

Horse - Bones of the thoracic limb (Left) (Lateral view

1. Cranial border
2. Scapula
3. Neck of scapula
4. Supraglenoid tubercle
5. Ventral angle
6. Infraglenoid tubercle
7. Shoulder joint
8. Lesser tubercle
9. Head of humerus
10. Greater tubercle
11. Intertubercular groove
12. Surface of infraspinous muscle
13. Neck of humerus
14. Tricipital muscle line
15. Body [Shaft] of humerus
16. Humerus
17. Condyle of humerus
18. Head
19. Neck of radius
20. Radius
21. Radiocarpal joint
22. Intercarpal joints
23. Carpometacarpal joints
24. Metacarpal IV
25. Metacarpal III
26. Metacarpophalangeal joints
27. Proximal interphalangeal joint
 [Pastern joint; PIP joint]
28. Distal interphalangeal joint
 [Coffin joint; DIP joint]
29. Cranial angle
30. Cartilage of scapula
31. Dorsal border
32. Supraspinous fossa
33. Caudal angle
34. Lateral surface
35. Tubercle of spine of scapula
36. Caudal border
37. Infraspinous fossa
38. Lateral supracondylar crest
39. Olecranon fossa
40. Olecranon tuber
41. Lateral epicondyle
42. Anconeal process
43. Olecranon
44. Humeroulnar joint
45. Elbow joint
46. Ulna
47. Lateral coronoid process
48. Humeroradial joint
49. Antebrachial interosseous space
50. Body [Shaft] of ulna
51. Accessory carpal bone [Pisiform]

Horse - Bones of the thoracic limb (Left) (Medial view)

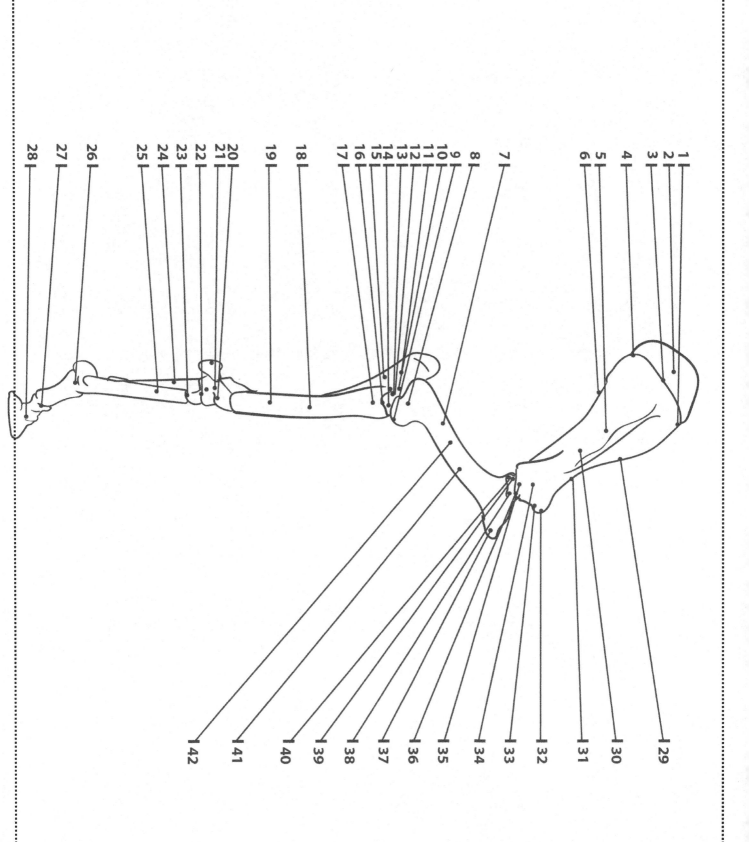

Horse - Bones of the thoracic limb (Left) (Medial view)

1. Cranial angle
2. Cartilage of scapula
3. Dorsal border
4. Caudal angle
5. Costal surface [Medial]
6. Caudal border
7. Humerus
8. Medial epicondyle
9. Condyle of humerus
10. Humeroulnar joint
11. Olecranon
12. Elbow joint
13. Medial coronoid process
14. Humeroradial joint
15. Ulna
16. Head
17. Neck of radius
18. Body [Shaft] of radius
19. Radius
20. Trochlea of radius
21. Radiocarpal joint
22. Intercarpal joints
23. Carpometacarpal joints
24. Metacarpal II
25. Metacarpal III
26. Metacarpophalangeal joints
27. Proximal interphalangeal joint
   [Pastern joint; PIP joint]
28. Distal interphalangeal joint
   [Coffin joint; DIP joint]

29. Cranial border
30. Scapula
31. Scapular notch
32. Supraglenoid tubercle
33. Coracoid process
34. Neck of scapula
35. Head of humerus
36. Ventral angle
37. Lesser tubercle
38. Neck of humerus
39. Shoulder joint
40. Infraglenoid tubercle
41. Tuberosity for teres major
42. Body [Shaft] of humerus

Horse - Scapula (Left) (Lateral view)

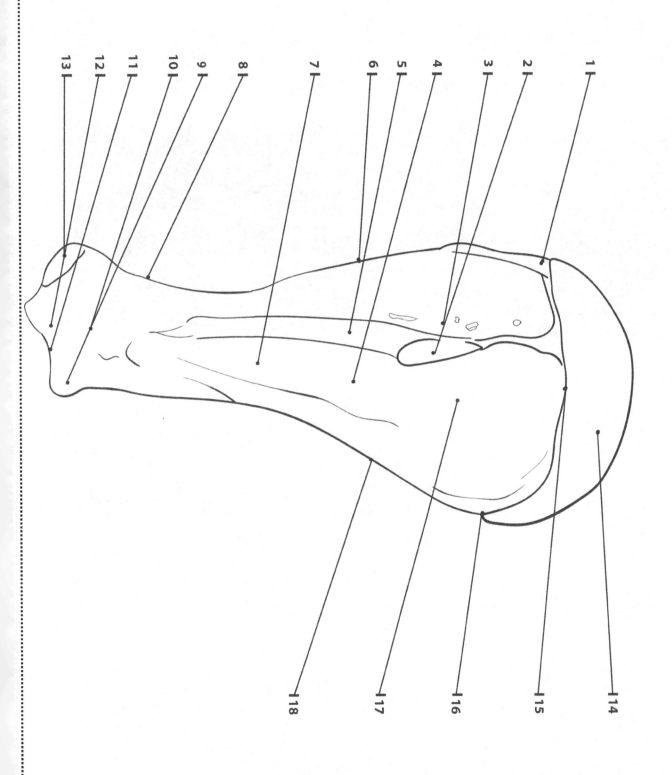

Horse - Scapula (Left) (Lateral view)

1. Cranial angle
2. Tubercle of spine of scapula
3. Supraspinous fossa
4. Infraspinous fossa
5. Spine of scapula
6. Cranial border
7. Scapula
8. Scapular notch
9. Infraglenoid tubercle
10. Neck of scapula
11. Glenoid cavity
12. Ventral angle
13. Supraglenoid tubercle
14. Cartilage of scapula
15. Dorsal border
16. Caudal angle
17. Lateral surface
18. Caudal border

Horse - Scapula (Left) (Medial view)

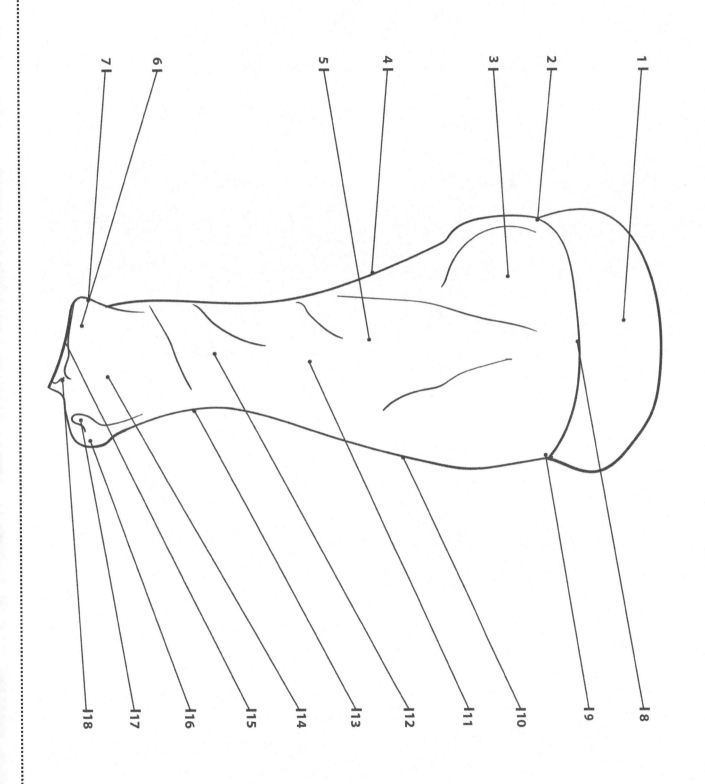

Horse - Scapula (Left) (Medial view)

1. Cartilage of scapula
2. Caudal angle
3. Facies serrata
4. Caudal border
5. Costal surface [Medial]
6. Ventral angle
7. Infraglenoid tubercle
8. Dorsal border
9. Cranial angle
10. Cranial border
11. Subscapular fossa
12. Scapula
13. Scapular notch
14. Neck of scapula
15. Glenoid cavity
16. Supraglenoid tubercle
17. Coracoid process
18. Glenoid notch

Horse - Scapula (Left) (Cranial view)

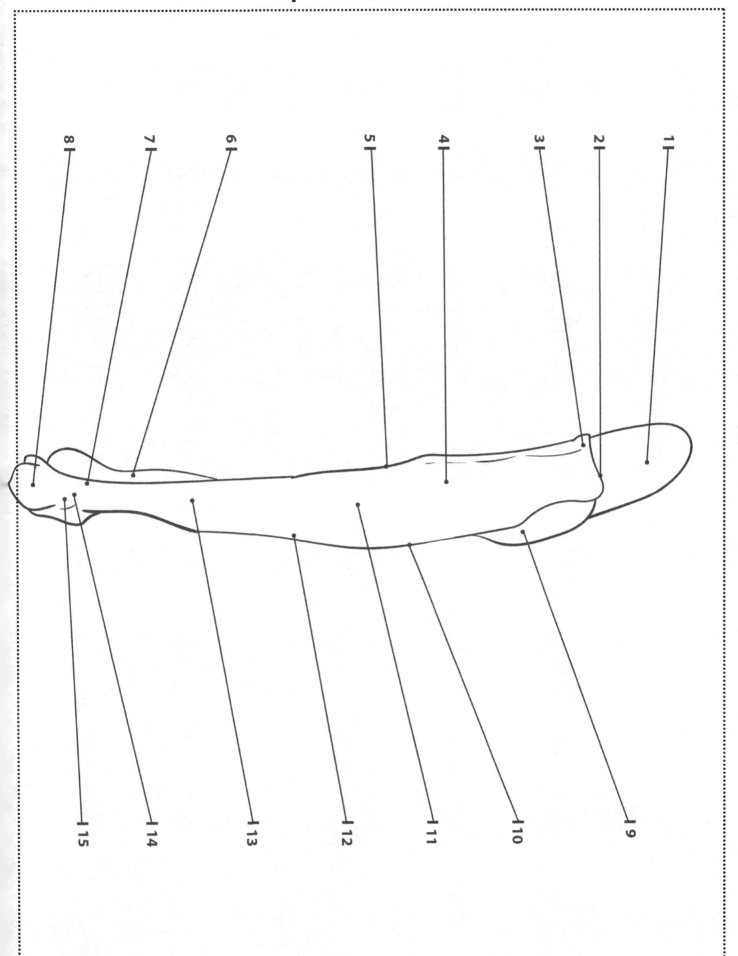

Horse - Scapula (Left) (Cranial view)

1. Cartilage of scapula
2. Dorsal border
3. Cranial angle
4. Lateral surface
5. Cranial border
6. Costal surface [Medial]
7. Scapular notch
8. Supraglenoid tubercle
9. Infraspinous fossa
10. Tubercle of spine of scapula
11. Supraspinous fossa
12. Spine of scapula
13. Scapula
14. Neck of scapula
15. Ventral angle

Horse - Scapula (Left) (Caudalview)

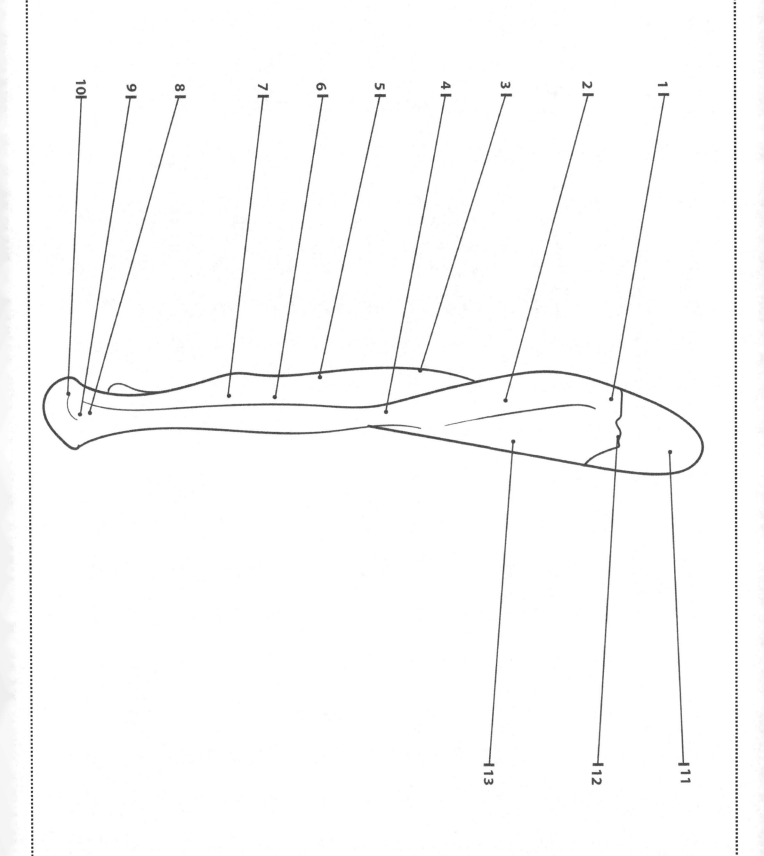

Horse - Scapula (Left) (Caudalview)

1. Caudal angle
2. Scapula
3. Tubercle of spine of scapula
4. Caudal border
5. Spine of scapula
6. Infraspinous fossa
7. Lateral surface
8. Neck of scapula
9. Ventral angle
10. Infraglenoid tubercle
11. Cartilage of scapula
12. Dorsal border
13. Costal surface [Medial]

Horse - Scapula (Left) (Distal view)

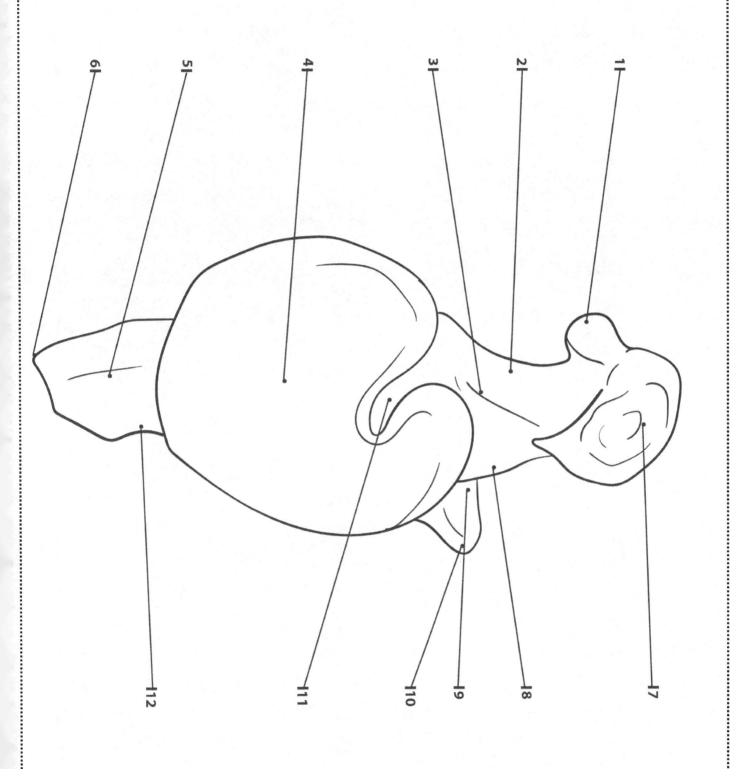

Horse - Scapula (Left) (Distal view)

1. Coracoid process
2. Costal surface [Medial]
3. Neck of scapula
4. Glenoid cavity
5. Scapula
6. Caudal border
7. Supraglenoid tubercle
8. Lateral surface
9. Supraspinous fossa
10. Spine of scapula
11. Glenoid notch
12. Infraspinous fossa

Horse - Humerus (Left) (Lateral view)

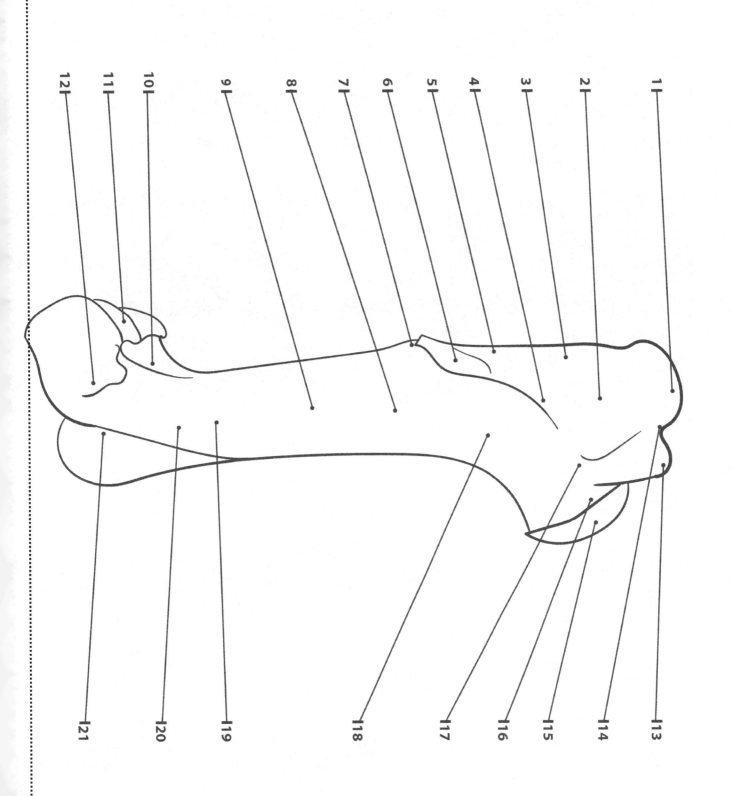

Horse - Humerus (Left) (Lateral view)

1. Cranial part of greater tubercle
2. Surface of infraspinous muscle
3. Crest of greater tubercle
4. Tricipital muscle line
5. Cranial surface
6. Deltoid tuberosity
7. Humeral crest
8. Body [Shaft] of humerus
9. Lateral surface
10. Radial fossa
11. Condyle of humerus
12. Lateral epicondyle
13. Caudal part of greater tubercle
14. Greater tubercle
15. Head of humerus
16. Neck of humerus
17. Tuberosity for teres minor
18. Humerus
19. Groove of brachialis
20. Lateral supracondylar crest
21. Olecranon fossa

Horse - Humerus (Left) (Medial view)

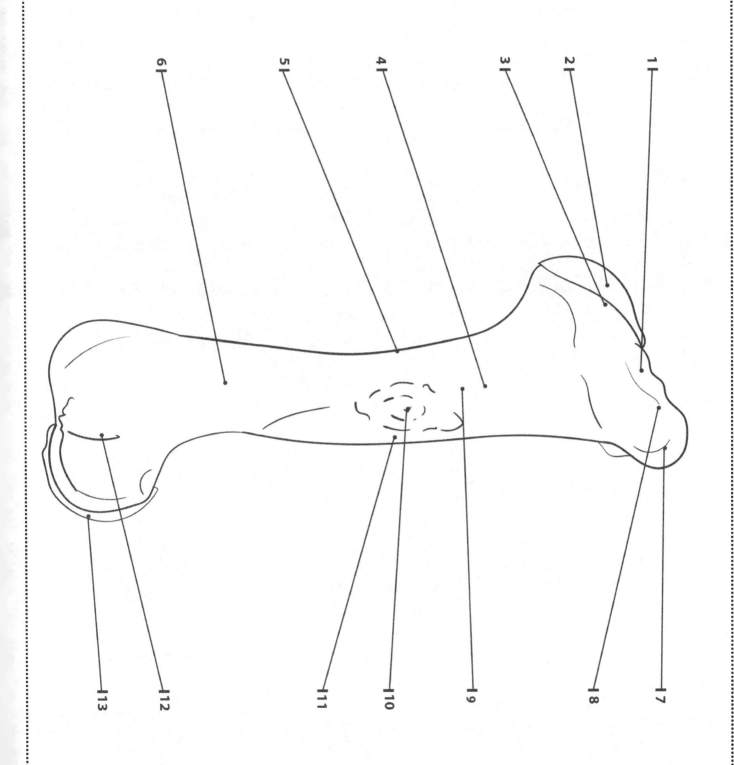

Horse - Humerus (Left) (Medial view)

1. Caudal part of lesser tubercle
2. Head of humerus
3. Neck of humerus
4. Body [Shaft] of humerus
5. Caudal surface
6. Humerus
7. Cranial part of lesser tubercle
8. Lesser tubercle
9. Medial surface
10. Tuberosity for teres major
11. Cranial surface
12. Medial epicondyle
13. Condyle of humerus

Horse - Humerus (Left) (Cranial view)

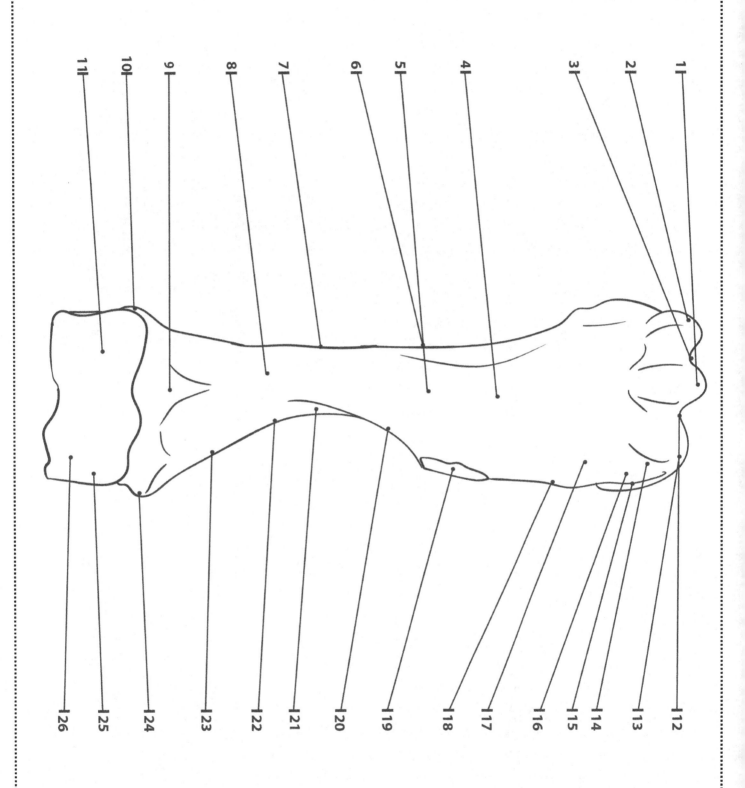

Horse - Humerus (Left) (Lateral view)

1. Intermediate tubercle
2. Cranial part of lesser tubercle
3. Intertubercular groove
4. Body [Shaft] of humerus
5. Cranial surface
6. Tuberosity for teres major
7. Medial surface
8. Humerus
9. Radial fossa
10. Medial epicondyle
11. Trochlea of humerus
12. Intertubercular groove
13. Cranial part of greater tubercle
14. Greater tubercle
15. Neck of humerus
16. Surface of infraspinous muscle
17. Crest of greater tubercle
18. Tricipital muscle line
19. Deltoid tuberosity
20. Humeral crest
21. Lateral surface
22. Groove of brachialis Lateral
23. supracondylar crest
24. Lateral epicondyle
25. Capitulum of humerus
26. Condyle of humerus

Horse - Humerus (Left) (Caudal view)

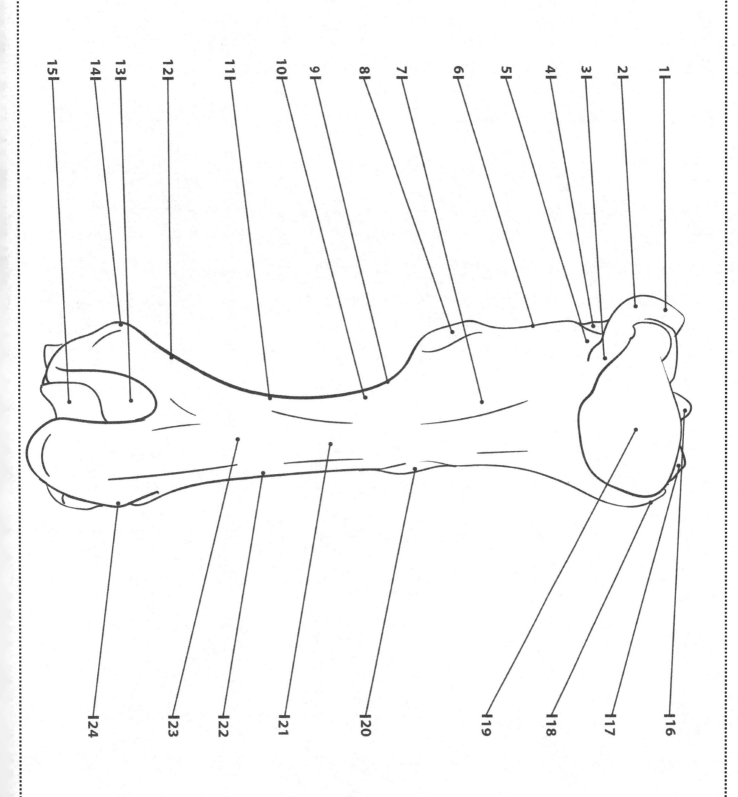

Horse - Humerus (Left) (Caudal view)

1. Caudal part of greater tubercle
2. Greater tubercle
3. Neck of humerus
4. Surface of infraspinous muscle
5. Tuberosity for teres minor
6. Tricipital muscle line
7. Body [Shaft] of humerus
8. Deltoid tuberosity
9. Humeral crest
10. Groove of brachialis
11. Lateral surface
12. Lateral supracondylar crest
13. Olecranon fossa
14. Lateral epicondyle
15. Trochlea of humerus

16. Intermediate tubercle
17. Cranial part of lesser tubercle
18. Caudal part of lesser tubercle
19. Head of humerus
20. Tuberosity for teres major
21. Caudal surface
22. Medial surface
23. Humerus
24. Medial epicondyle

Horse - Humerus (Left) (Proximal view)

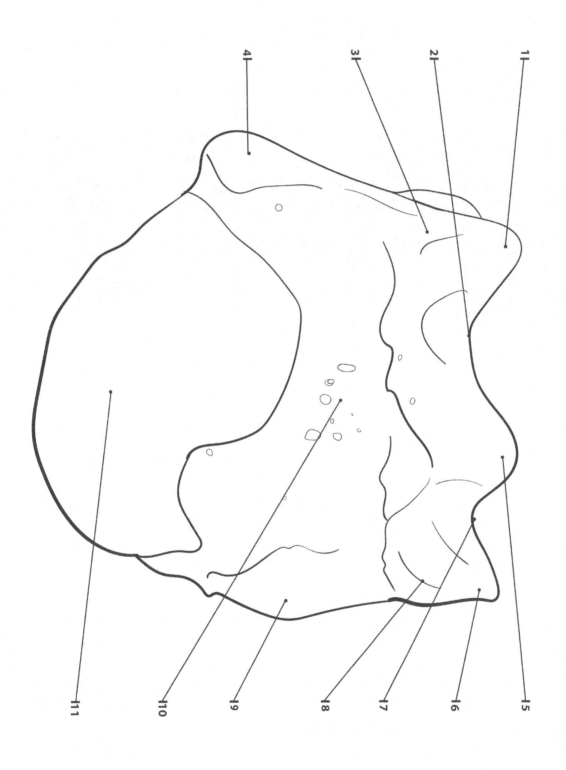

Horse - Humerus (Left) (Proximal view)

1. Cranial part of greater tubercle
2. Intertubercular groove
3. Greater tubercle
4. Caudal part of greater tubercle
5. Intermediate tubercle
6. Cranial part of lesser tubercle
7. Intertubercular groove
8. Lesser tubercle
9. Caudal part of lesser tubercle
10. Humerus
11. Head of humerus

Horse - Humerus (Left) (Distal view)

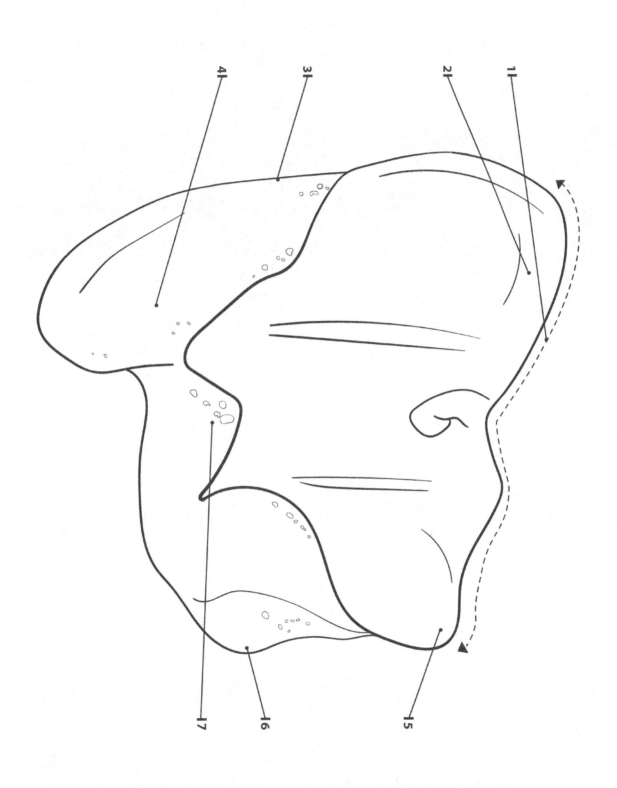

Horse - Humerus (Left) (Distal view)

1. Condyle of humerus
2. Trochlea of humerus
3. Medial epicondyle
4. Humerus

5. Capitulum of humerus
6. Lateral epicondyle
7. Olecranon fossa

Horse - Radius / Ulna (Left) (Lateral view)

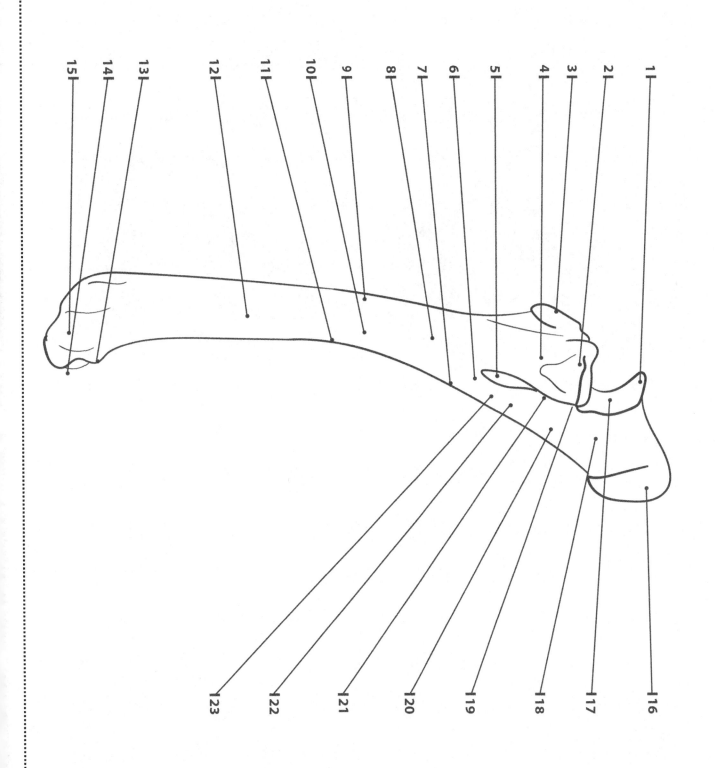

Horse - Radius / Ulna (Left) (Lateral view)

1. Anconeal process
2. Head
3. Radial tuberosity
4. Neck of radius
5. Antebrachial interosseous space
6. Lateral margin
7. Caudal border
8. Lateral margin
9. Cranial surface
10. Body [shaft] of radius
11. Caudal surface
12. Radius
13. Transverse crest
14. Trochlea of radius
15. Lateral styloid process

16. Olecranon tuber
17. Trochlear notch
18. Olecranon
19. Lateral coronoid process
20. Ulna
21. Proximal radioulnar joint
22. Body [Shaft] of ulna
23. Lateral surface

Horse - Radius / Ulna (Left) (Medial view)

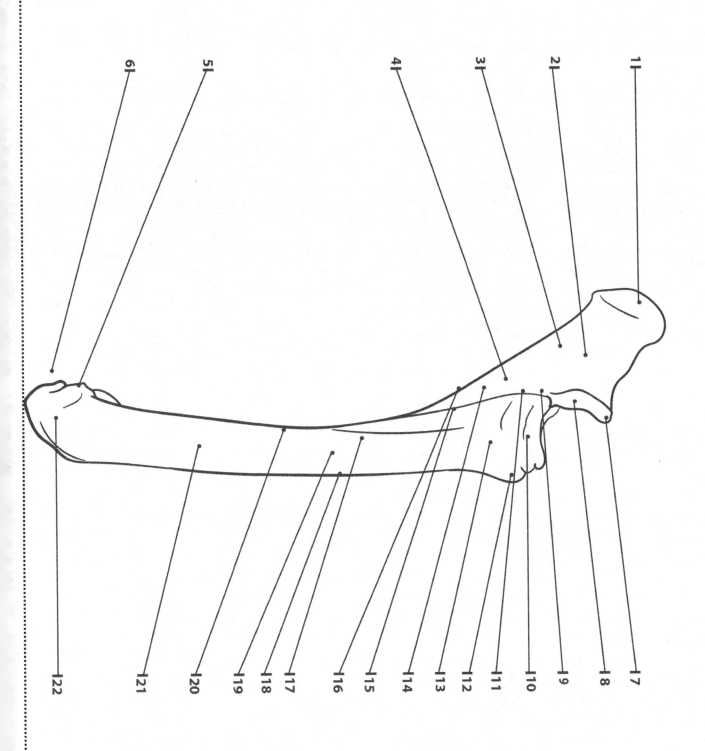

Horse - Radius / Ulna (Left) (Medial view)

1. Olecranon tuber
2. Olecranon
3. Ulna
4. Medial surface
5. Transverse crest
6. Trochlea of radius
7. Anconeal process
8. Trochlear notch
9. Medial coronoid process
10. Head
11. Proximal radioulnar joint
12. Radial tuberosity
13. Neck of radius
14. Body [Shaft] of ulna
15. Antebrachial interosseous space
16. Caudal border
17. Medial margin
18. Cranial surface
19. Body [Shaft] of radius
20. Caudal surface
21. Radius
22. Medial styloid process

Horse - Radius / Ulna (Left) (Medial view)

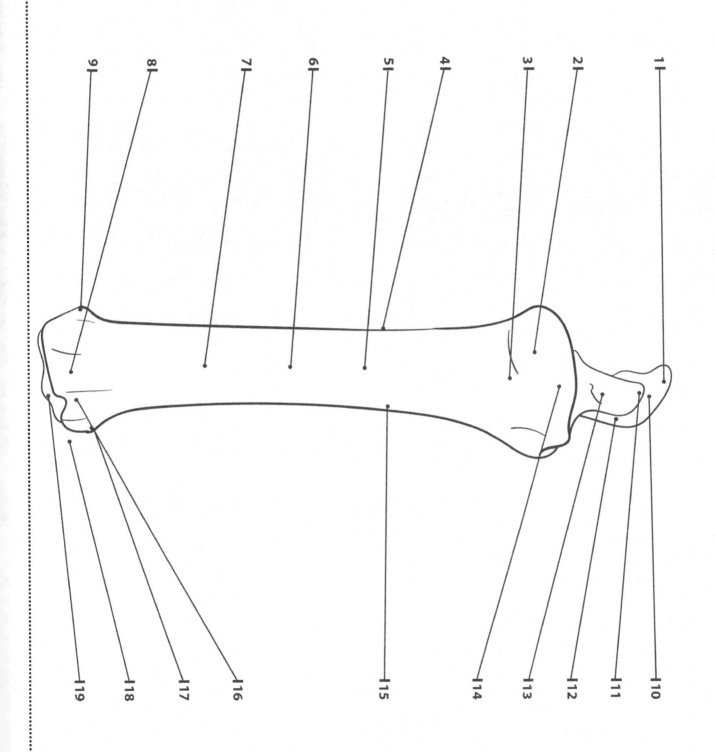

Horse - Radius / Ulna (Left) (Medial view)

1. Olecranon tuber
2. Radial tuberosity
3. Neck of radius
4. Medial margin
5. Body [shaft] of radius
6. Cranial surface
7. Radius
8. Groove of extensor carpi radialis
9. Medial styloid process
10. Olecranon
11. Anconeal process
12. Ulna
13. Trochlear notch
14. Head
15. Lateral margin
16. Groove of extensor digitali communis
17. Lateral styloid process
18. Trochlea of radius
19. Carpal articular surface

Horse - Ulna (Left) (Cranial view)

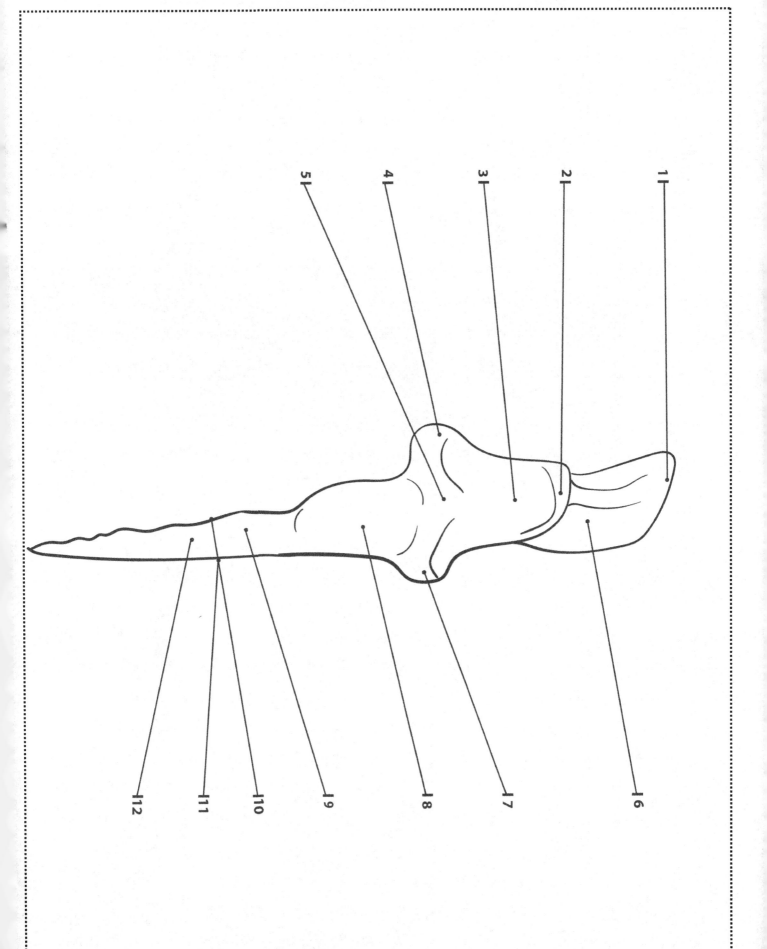

Horse - Ulna (Left) (Cranial view)

1. Olecranon tuber
2. Anconeal process
3. Trochlear notch
4. Lateral coronoid process
5. Radial notch
6. Olecranon
7. Medial coronoid process
8. Ulna
9. Body [Shaft] of ulna
10. Medial margin
11. Lateral margin
12. Cranial surface

Horse - Radius / Ulna (Left) (Caudal view)

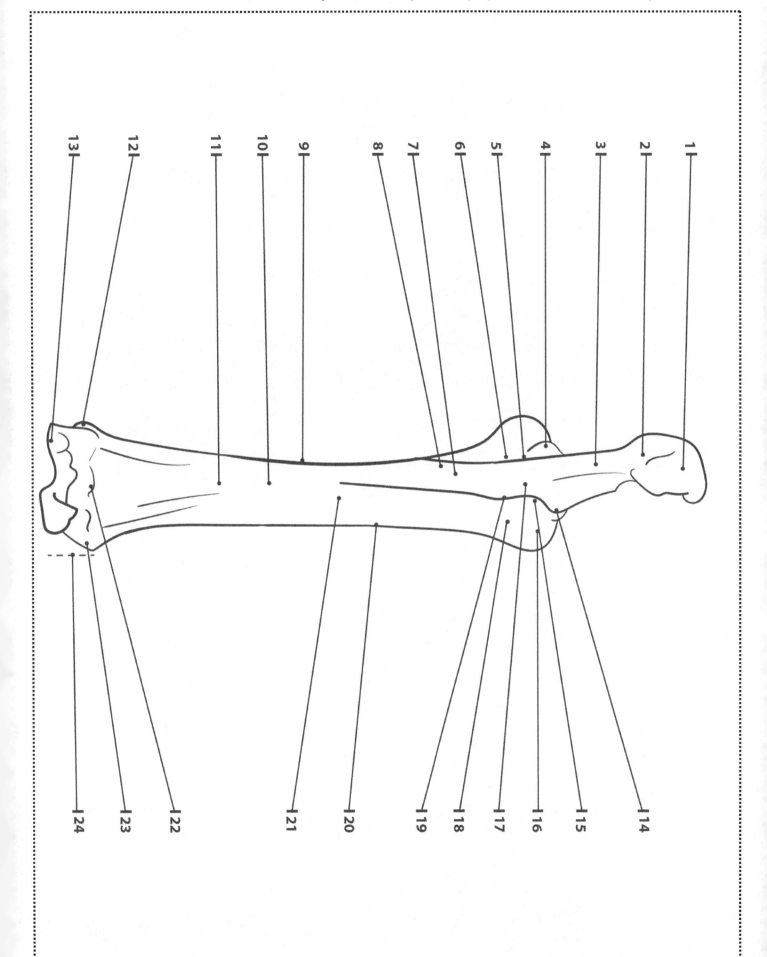

Horse - Radius / Ulna (Left) (Caudal view)

1. Olecranon tuber
2. Ulna
3. Olecranon
4. Lateral coronoid process
5. Lateral surface
6. Lateral margin
7. Body [Shaft] of ulna
8. Caudal border
9. Lateral margin
10. Caudal surface
11. Radius
12. Lateral styloid process
13. Carpal anicular surface
14. Medial coronoid process
15. Proximal radioulnar joint
16. Head
17. Medial surface
18. Neck of radius
19. Medial margin
20. Medial margin
21. Body [Shaft] of radius
22. Transverse crest
23. Medial styloid process
24. Trochlea of radius

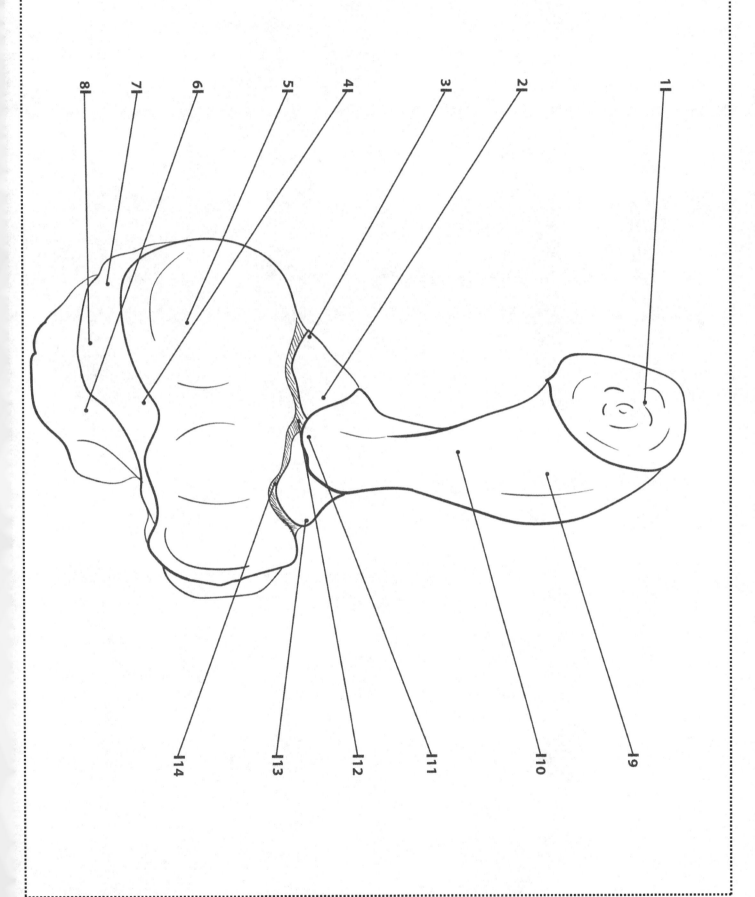

Horse - Radius / Ulna (Left) (Proximal view)

1. Olecranon tuber
2. Trochlear notch
3. Medial coronoid process
4. Head
5. Articular fovea of radial head
6. Body [Shaft] of radius
7. Radius
8. Radial tuberosity
9. Ulna
10. Olecranon
11. Anconeal process
12. Radial notch
13. Lateral coronoid process
14. Proximal radioulnar joint

Horse - Radius / Ulna (Left) (Distal view)

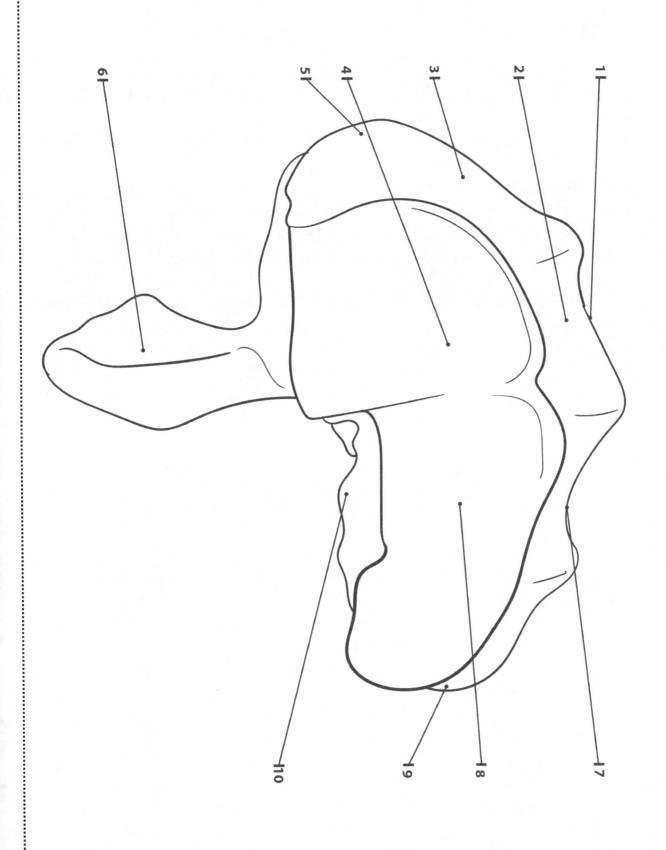

Horse - Radius / Ulna (Left) (Distal view)

1. Groove of extensor carpi radialis
2. Radius
3. Ulna
4. Trochlea of radius
5. Medial styloid process
6. Olecranon

7. Groove of extensor digitali communis
8. Carpal articular surface
9. Lateral styloid process
10. Transverse crest

Horse - Carpus (Left) (Lateral view)

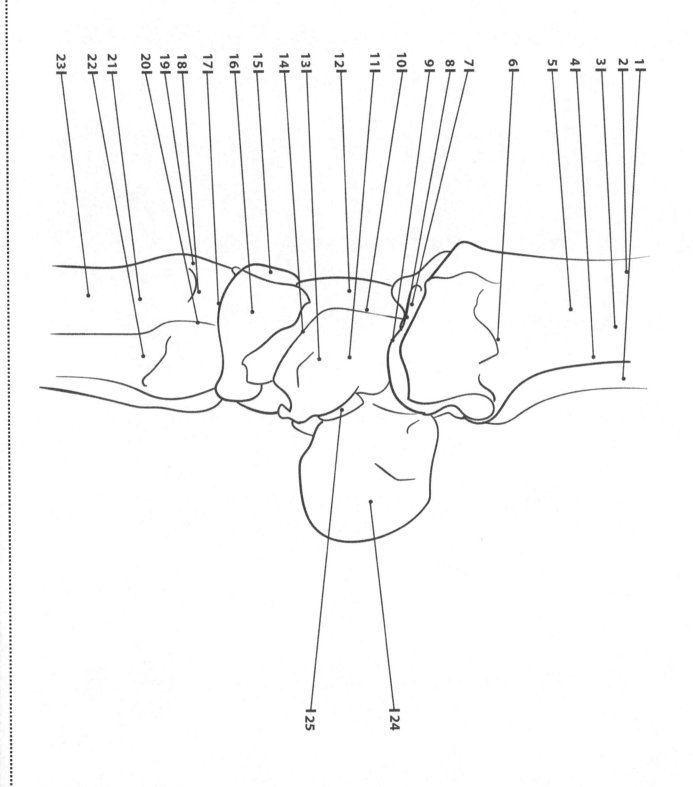

Horse - Carpus (Left) (Lateral view)

1. Caudal surface
2. Cranial surface
3. Body [Shaft] of radius
4. Lateral margin
5. Radius
6. Lateral styloid process
7. Trochlea of radius
8. Carpal articular surface
9. Radiocarpal joint
10. Intercarpal joints
11. Ulnar carpal bone [Triquetrum]
12. Intermediate carpal bone [Lunatum]
13. Carpal bones
14. Mediocarpal join
15. Carpal bone Ill [Capitatum]
16. Carpal bone IV [Hamatum
17. Carpometacarpal joints
18. Base
19. Tuberosity of metacarpal II
20. Intermetacarpal joints
21. Metacarpal II
22. Metacarpal IV
23. Body

23..Accessory carpal bone [Pisiform]
24..Joint of accessory carpal bone

Horse - Carpus (Left) (Medial view)

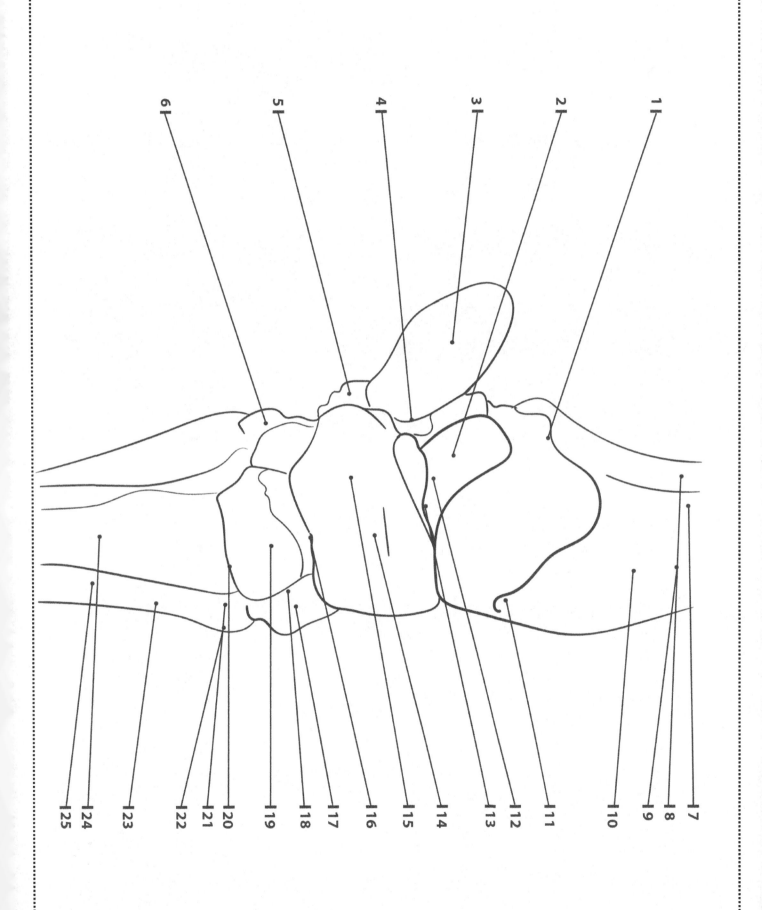

Horse - Carpus (Left) (Medial view)

1. Transverse crest
2. Trochlea of radius
3. Accessory carpal bone [Pisiform]
4. Joint of accessory carpal bone
5. Intermediate carpal bone [Lunatum]
6. Carpal bone IV [Hamatum]
7. Medial margin
8. Caudal surface
9. Body [Shaft] of radius
10. Radius
11. Medial styloid process
12. Carpal articular surface
13. Radiocarpal joint
14. Radial carpal bone [Scaphoid]
15. Carpal bones
16. Mediocarpal joint
17. Carpal bone III [Capitatum]
18. Intercarpal joints
19. Carpal bone II [Trapézoid]
20. Carpometacarpal joints
21. Base
22. Tuberosity of metacarpal Ill
23. Metacarpal III
24. Metacarpal II
25. Body

Horse - Carpus (Left) (Dorsal view)

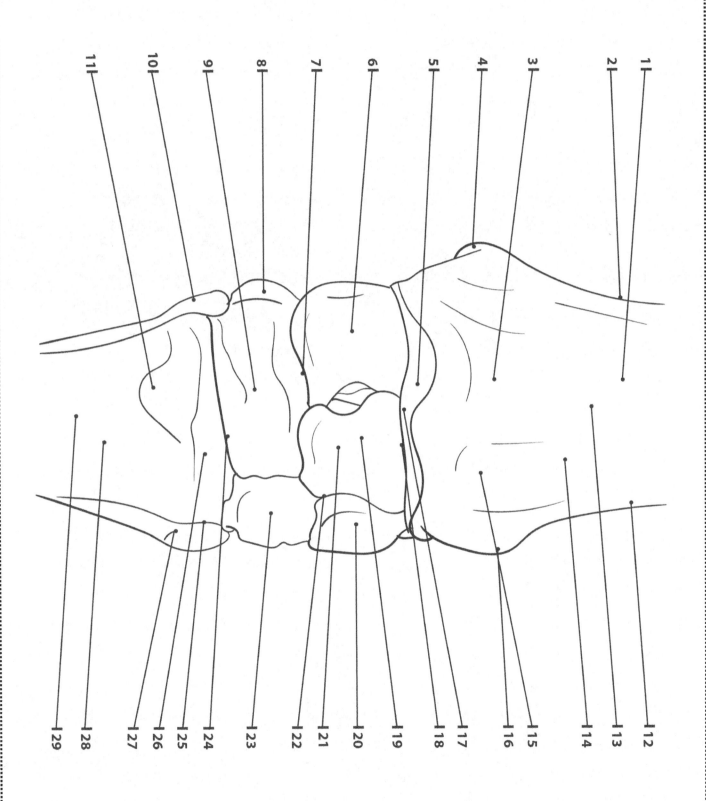

Horse - Carpus (Left) (Dorsal view)

1. Body [Shaft] of radius
2. Medial margin
3. Groove of extensor carpi radialis
4. Medial styloid process
5. Trochlea of radius
6. Radial carpal bone [Scaphoid]
7. Mediocarpal joint
8. Carpal bone II [Trapézoid]
9. Carpal bone Ill [Capitatum]
10. Metacarpal II
11. Tuberosity of metacarpal Ill
12. Lateral margin
13. Cranial surface
14. Radius
15. Groove of extensor digitali communis
16. Lateral styloid process
17. Carpal articular surface
18. Radiocarpal joint
19. Intermediate carpal bone [Lunatum]
20. Ulnar carpal bone [Triquetrum]
21. Carpal bones
22. Intercarpal joints
23. Carpal bone IV [Hamatum]
24. Carpometacarpal joints
25. Intermetacarpal joints
26. Base
27. Metacarpal IV
28. Metacarpal Ill
29. Body

Horse - Carpus (Left) (Palmar view)

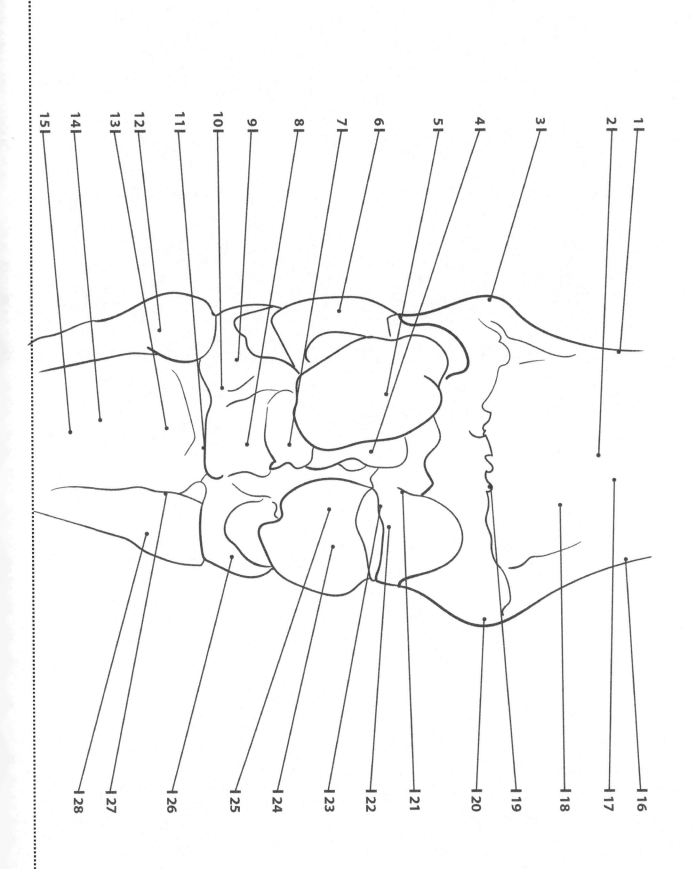

Horse - Carpus (Left) (Palmar view)

1. Lateral margin
2. Caudal surface
3. Lateral styloid process
4. Intermediate carpal bone [Lunatum]
5. Accessory carpal bone [Pisiform]
6. Ulnar carpal bone [Triquetrum]
7. Mediocarpal joint
8. Carpal bone III [Capitatum]
9. Carpal bone IV [Hamatum]
10. Intercarpal joints
11. Carpometacarpal joints
12. Metacarpal IV
13. Base
14. Metacarpal III
15. Body
16. Medial margin
17. Body [Shaft] of radius
18. Radius
19. Transverse crest
20. Medial styloid process
21. Trochlea of radius
22. Carpal articular surface
23. Radiocarpal joint
24. Radial carpal bone [Scaphoid]
25. Carpal bones
26. Carpal bone II [Trapézoid]
27. Intermetacarpal joint
28. Metacarpal II

Horse - Metacarpals (Left) (Lateral view)

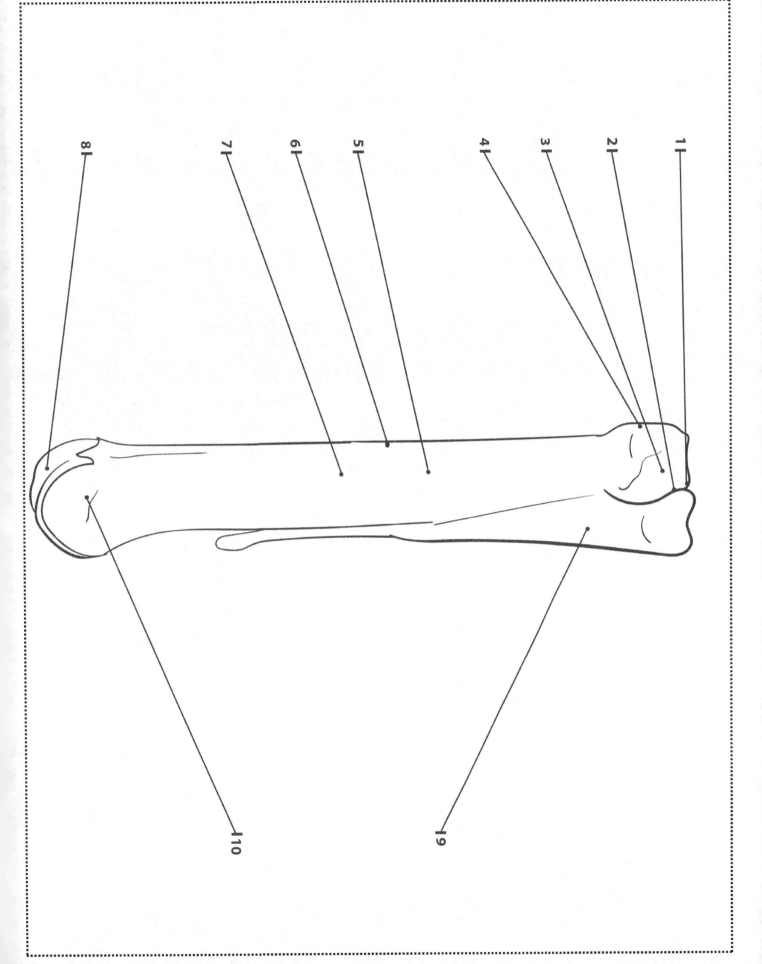

Horse - Metacarpals (Left) (Lateral view)

1. Articular surface
2. Intermetacarpal joints
3. Base
4. Tuberosity of metacarpal Ill
5. Metacarpal Ill
6. Dorsal surface
7. Body
8. Trochlea of metacarpal
9. Metacarpal IV
10. Head

Horse - Metacarpals (Left) (Medial view)

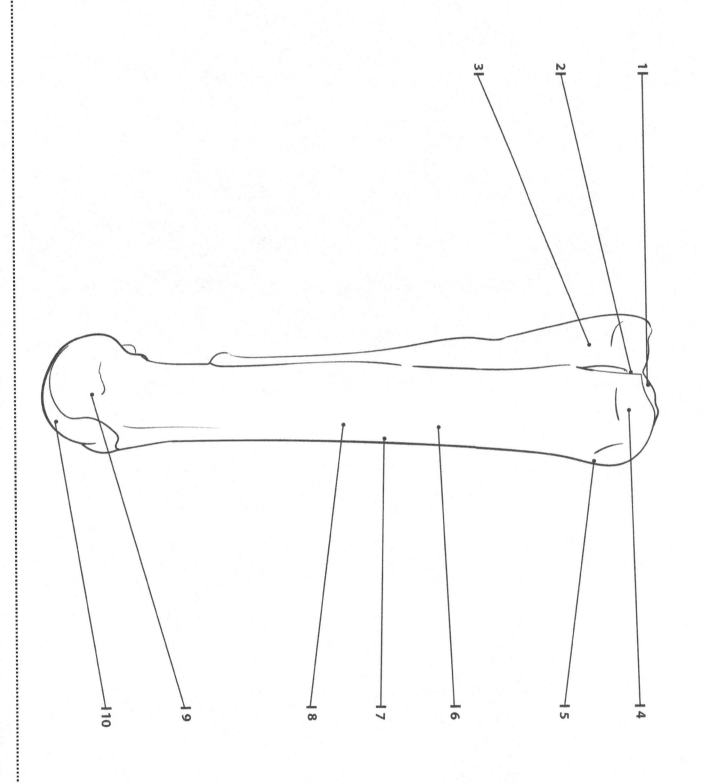

Horse - Metacarpals (Left) (Medial view)

1. Articular surface
2. Intermetacarpal joints
3. Metacarpal II
4. Base
5. Tuberosity of metacarpal III
6. Metacarpal III
7. Dorsal surface
8. Body
9. Head
10. Trochlea of metacarpal

Horse - Metacarpals (Left) (Dorsal view)

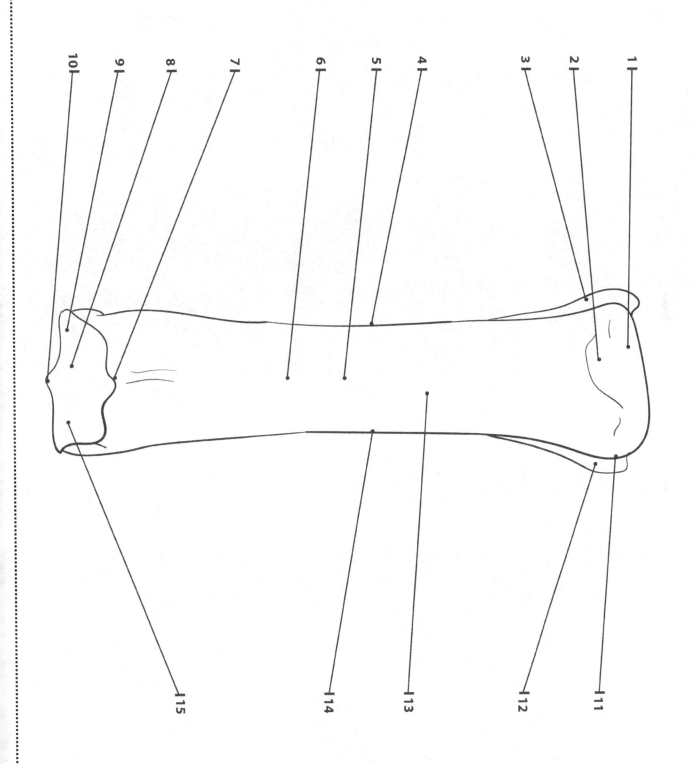

Horse - Metacarpals (Left) (Dorsal view)

1. Base
2. Tuberosity of metacarpal III
3. Metacarpal ll
4. Medial margin
5. Body
6. Dorsal surface
7. Head
8. Trochlea of metacarpal
9. Medial condyle
10. Sagittal crest
11. Intermetacarpal joints
12. Metacarpal IV
13. Metacarpal lll
14. Lateral margin
15. Lateral condyle

Horse - Metacarpals (Left) (Palmar view)

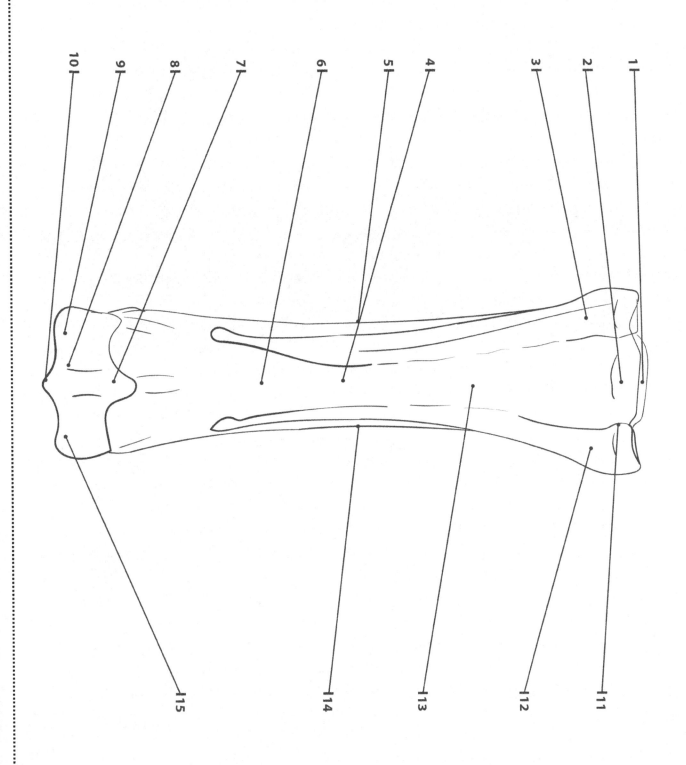

Horse - Metacarpals (Left) (Palmar view)

1. Articular surface
2. Base
3. Metacarpal IV
4. Body
5. Lateral margin
6. Palmar surface
7. Head
8. Trochlea of metacarpal
9. Lateral condyle
10. Sagittal crest
11. Intermetacarpal joints
12. Metacarpal II
13. Metacarpal III
14. Medial margin
15. Medial condyle

Horse - Metacarpals (Left) (Proximal view)

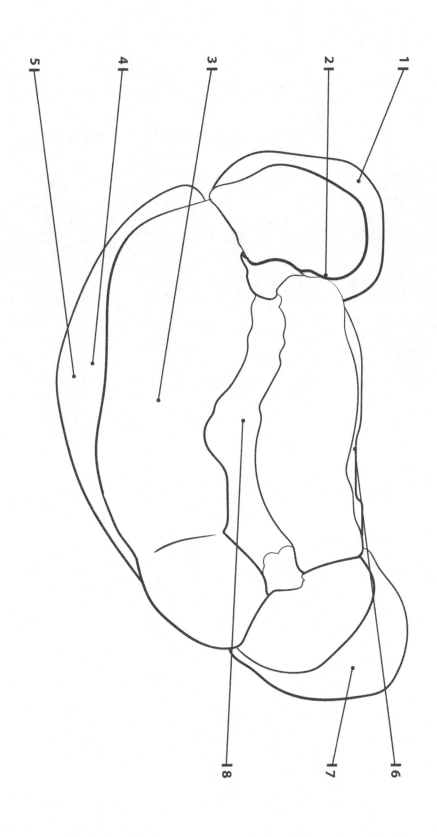

Horse - Metacarpals (Left) (Proximal view)

1. Metacarpal II
2. Intermetacarpal joints
3. Articular surface
4. Base
5. Tuberosity of metacarpal III
6. Palmar surface
7. Metacarpal IV
8. Metacarpal III

Horse - Metacarpal III (Left) (Distal view)

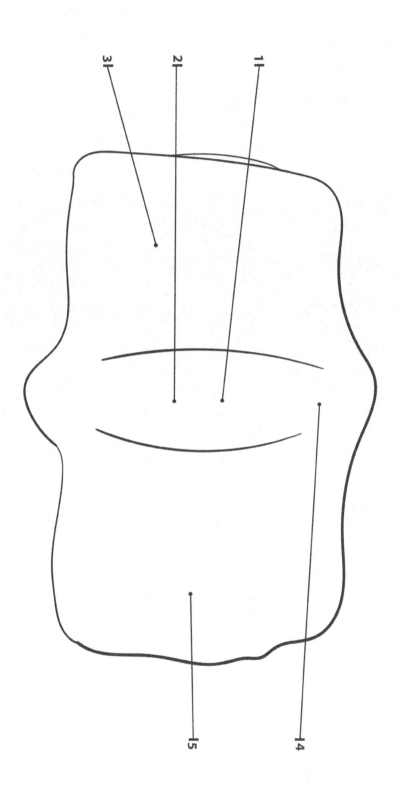

Horse - Metacarpal III (Left) (Distal view)

1. Sagittal crest
2. Metacarpal Ill
3. Medial condyle
4. Trochlea of metacarpal
5. Lateral condyle

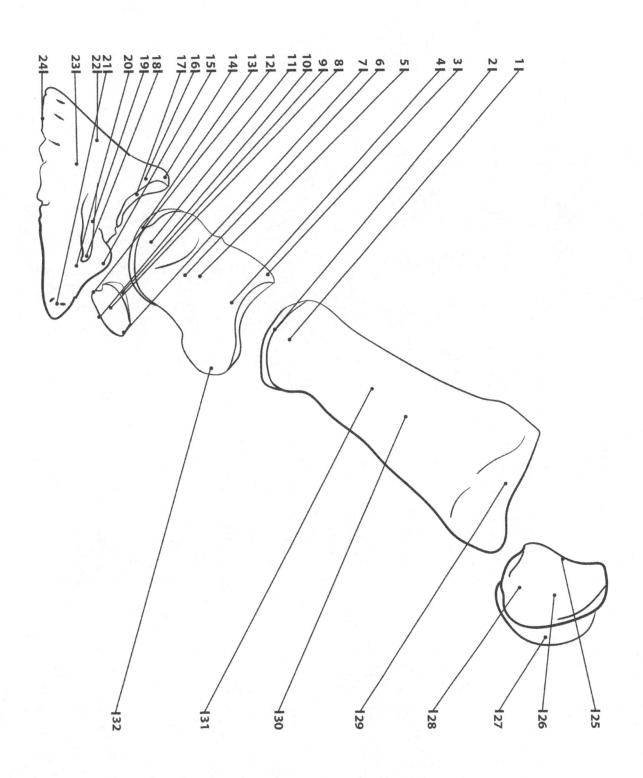

Horse - Digital bones of the hand (Left) (Lateral view)

1. Head of proximal phalanx
2. Lateral part of distal condyle of proximal phalanx
3. Extensor process
4. Base of middle phalanx
5. Middle phalanx [Short pastern bone]
6. Body of middle phatanx
7. Proximal border
8. Distal sesamoid bone
9. Articular surface
10. Flexor surface
11. Head of middle phalanx
12. Distal border
13. Lateral part of distal condyle of middle phalanx
14. Extensor process
15. Proximal part of lateral palmar process
16. Coronary border
17. Articular surface
18. Foramen of lateral palmar process
19. Lateral parietal groove
20. Lateral palmar process
21. Distal part of lateral palmar process
22. Parietal surface
23. Distal phalanx [Ungual bone;Coffin bone; Pedal bone]
24. Solar border
25. Articular surface
26. Surface for interosseous muscle
27. Flexor surface
28. Proximal sesamoid bones
29. Base of proximal phalanx
30. Body of proximal phalanx
31. Proximal phalanx [Long pastern bone]
32. Flexor tuberosity

Horse - Digital bones of the hand (Left) (Sagittal cross section)

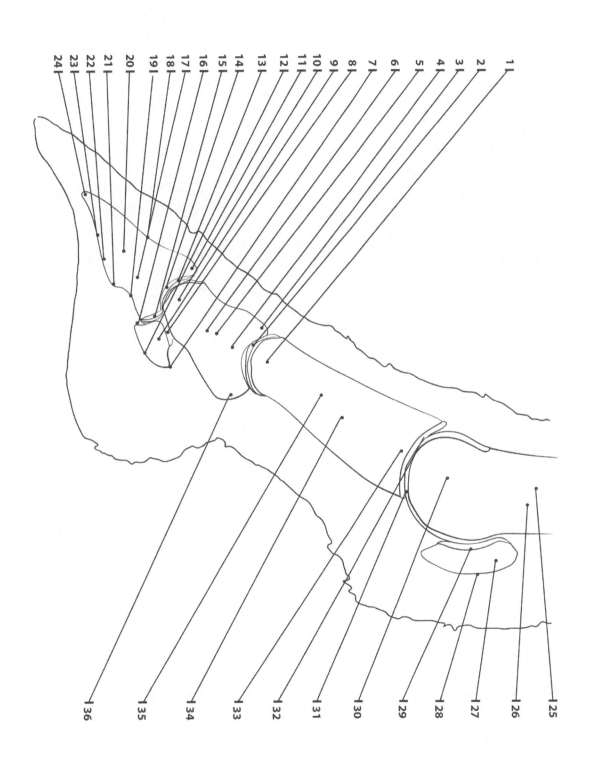

Horse - Digital bones of the hand (Left) (Sagittal cross section)

1. Head of proximal phalanx
2. Proxima interphalangeal joint [Paster joint; PIP joint]
3. Extensor process
4. Base of middle phalanx
5. Body of middle phalanx
6. Middle phalanx [Shor pester bone]
7. Proximal border
8. Articular surface
9. Distal sesamoid bone
10. Head of middle phalanx
11. Extensor process
12. Flexor surface
13. Distal interphalangeal jent [Coffin joint: DIP joint]
14. Articular surface
15. Articular surface of sesamoid
16. Distal border
17. Solar canal
18. Parietal surface
19. Flexor surface
20. Distal phalanx [Ungual bone: Coffin bone; Pedal bone]
21. Semilunar line
22. Cutaneous plane
23. Solar surface
24. Solar border
25. Body
26. Metacarpal Ill
27. Proximal sesamoid bones
28. Flexor surface
29. Articular surface
30. Head
31. Trochlea of metacarpal
32. Metacarpophalangeal joints
33. Base of proximal phalanx
34. Body of proximal phalanx
35. Proximal phalanx [Long pastembone]
36. Flexor tuberosity

Horse - Digital bones of the hand (Left) (Dorsal view)

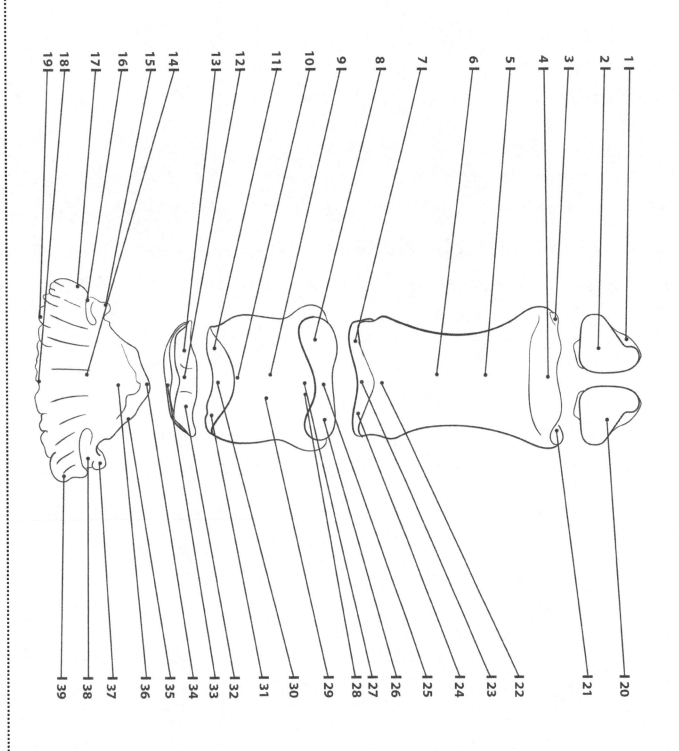

Horse - Digital bones of the hand (Left) (Dorsal view)

1. Surface foriferosseous muscle
2. Articular surface
3. Mediall part of glenoid cavity of proximal phalanx
4. Base of proximal phalanx
5. Body of proximal phalanx
6. Proximal phalanx [Long pastem bone]
7. Medial part of distal condyle of proximal phalanx
8. Mediall part of glenoid cavity of middle phalanx
9. Mile phalanx [Short pastern bone]
10. Head of middle phalanx
11. Medial part of distal condyle of middle phalanx
12. Sagittal ridge of distal sesamoid bone
13. Distal sesamoid bone
14. Parietal surface
15. Proximal part of medial palmar process
16. Medial parietal groove
17. Distal part of medial palmar process
18. Notch of solear border
19. Solar border
20. Proximal sesamoid bones
21. Lateral part of glenoid cavity of proximal phalanx
22. Head of proximal phalanx
23. Distal sagittal groove of proximal phalanx.
24. Lateral part of distal condyle of proximal phalanx
25. Sagittal ridge of base of middle phalanx
26. Lateral part of glenoid cavity of middle phalanx
27. Base of middle phalanx
28. Extensor process
29. Body of middle phalanx
30. Sagittal groove of middle phalanx
31. Lateral part of distal condyle of middle phalanx
32. Articular surface
33. Distal border
34. Extensor process
35. Coronary border
36. Distal phalanx [Ungual bone: Coffin bone; Pedal bone]
37. Proximal part of lateral palmer process
38. Lateral parietal groove
39. Distal part of lateral palmar process

Horse - Digital bones of the hand (Left) (Plantar view)

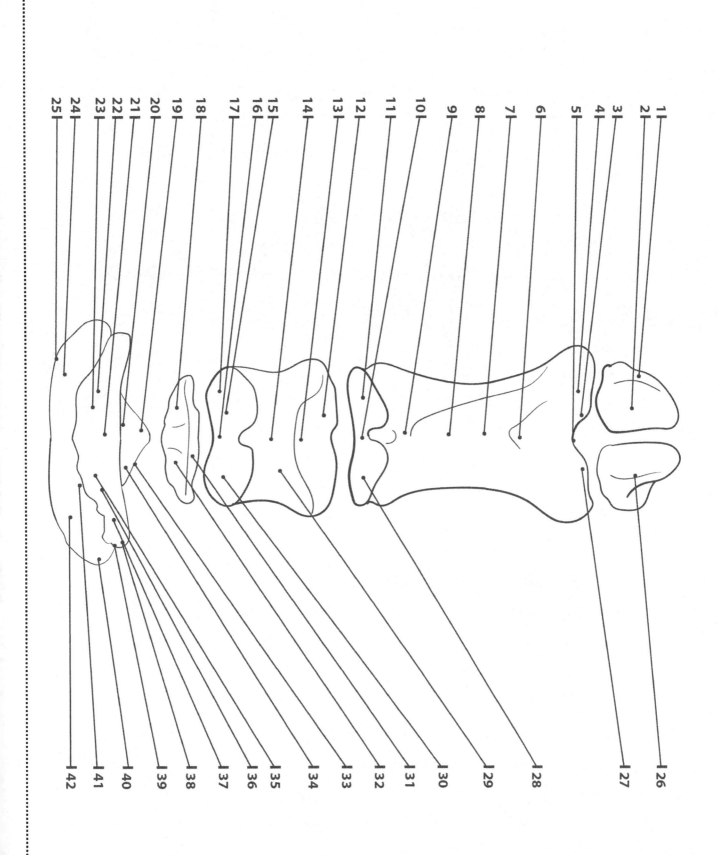

Horse - Digital bones of the hand (Left) (Plantar view)

1. Surface for interosseousmuscle
2. Flexor surface
3. Lateral palmar eminence
4. Base of proximal phalanx
5. Proximal sagittal groove of proximal phalanx
6. Body of proximal phalanx
7. Proximal phalanx [Long pastern bone]
8. Trigon of proximal phalanx
9. Head of proximal phalanx
10. Distal sagittal groove of proximal phalanx
11. Lateral part of distal condyle of proximal phalanx
12. Base of middle phalanx
13. Flexor tuberosity
14. Middle phalanx [Short pastern bone]
15. Head of middle phalanx
16. Sagittal groove of middle phalanx
17. Lateral part of distal condyle of middle phalanx
18. Distal sesamoid bone
19. Articular surface
20. Articular surface of sesamoid
21. Flexor surface
22. Lateral solear groove
23. Lateral solear foramen
24. Solar surface
25. Solar border
26. Proximal sesamoid bones
27. Medial palmar eminence
28. Medial part of distal condyle of proximal phalanx
29. Body of middle phalanx
30. Medial part of distal condyle of middle phalanx
31. Proximal border
32. Flexor surface
33. Coronary border
34. Mediall part of glenoid cavity of distal phalanx
35. Medial solear foramen
36. Medial solear groove
37. Distal phalanx [Ungual bone :Coffin bone; Pedal bone]
38. Proximal part of medial palmar process
39. Notch of medial palmar process
40. Distal part of medial palmar process
41. Semilunar line
42. Cutaneous plane

Horse - Digital bones of the hand (Left) (Proximal view)

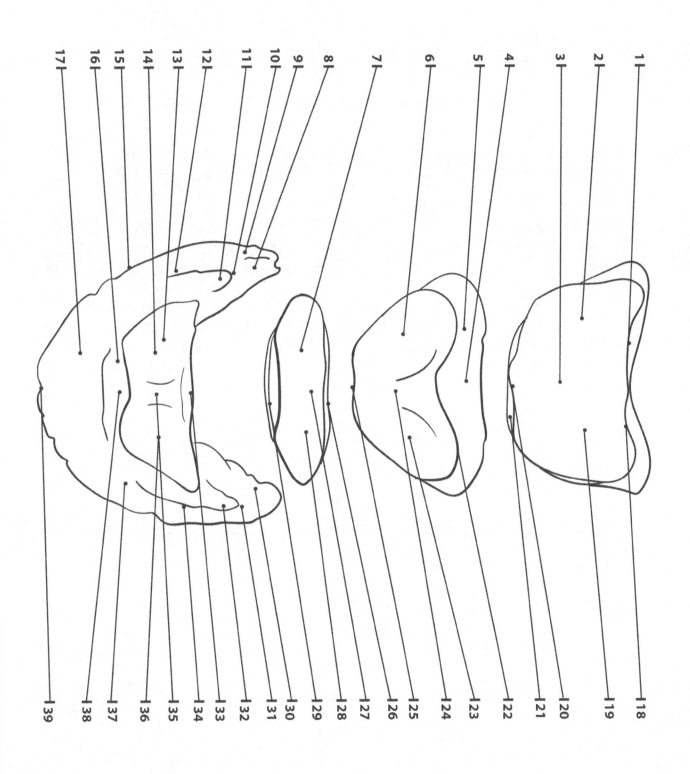

Horse - Digital bones of the hand (Left) (Proximal view)

1. Medial palmar eminence
2. Mediall part of glenoid cavity of proximal phalanx
3. Proximal sagittal groove of proximal phalanx
4. Flexor tuberosity
5. Middle phalanx [Short pastern bone]
6. Mediall part of glenoid cavity of middie phalanx
7. Distal sesamoid bone
8. Distal part of medial palmarprocess
9. Medial palmar process
10. Notch of medial palmar process
11. Proximal part of medial palmar process
12. Medial parietal groove
13. Mediall part of glenoid cavity of distal phalanx
14. Articular surface
15. Solar border
16. Coronary border
17. Parietal surface

18. Lateral palmar eminence
19. Lateral part of glenoid cavity of proximal phalanx
20. Proximal phalanx [Long pastern bone]
21. Base of proximal phalanx
22. Base of middle phalanx
23. Lateral part of glenoid cavity of middle phalanx
24. Sagittal ridge of base of middle phalanx
25. Extensor process
26. Proximal border
27. Sagittal ridge of distal sesamoid bone
28. Articular surface
29. Distal border
30. Lateral palmar process
31. Notch of lateral palmar process
32. Proximal part of lateral palmar process
33. Articular surface of sesamoid
34. Lateral parietal groove
35. Sagittal ridge of articular surface of distal phalanx
36. Lateral part of glenoid cavity of distal phalanx
37. Distal phalanx [Ungual bone;Coffin bone; Pedal bone]
38. Extensor process
39. Notch of solear border

Digital bones of the hand (Left) (Distal view)

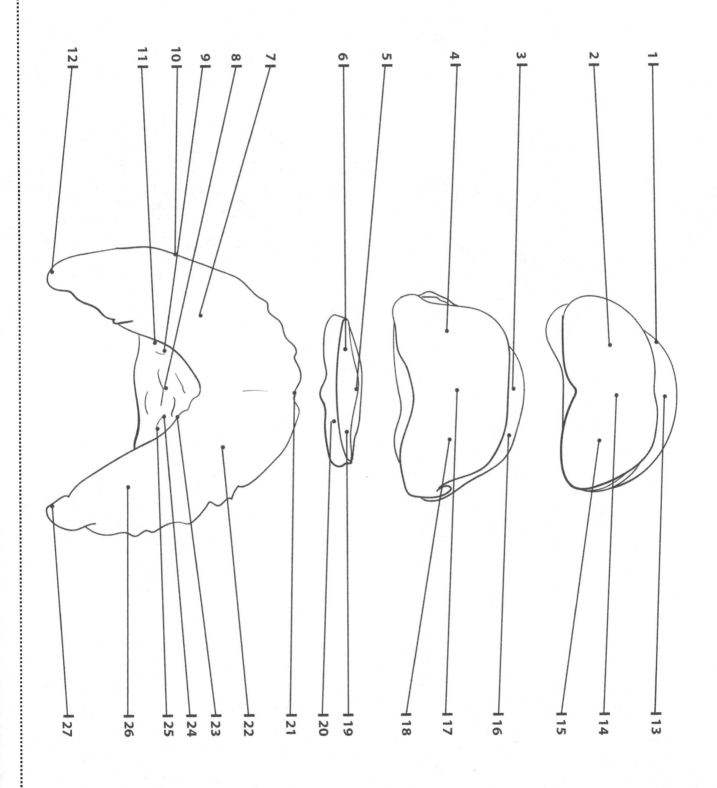

Digital bones of the hand (Left) (Distal view)

1. Proximal phalanx [Long pastern bone]
2. Medial part of distal condyle of proximal p
3. Middle phalanx [Short pastern bone]
4. Medial part of distal condyle of middle ph
5. Sagittal ridge of distal sesamoid bone
6. Distal sesamoid bone
7. Solar surface
8. Flexor surface
9. Medial solear foramen
10. Solar border
11. Medial solear groove
12. Distal part of medial palmar process

13. Head of proximal phalanx
14. Distal sagittal groove of proximal phalanx
15. Lateral part of distal condyle of proximal p
16. Head of middle phalanx
17. Sagittal groove of middle phalanx
18. Lateral part of distal condyle of middle ph
19. Articular surface
20. Distal border
21. Notch of solear border
22. Cutaneous plane
23. Semilunar line
24. Lateral solear foramen
25. Lateral solear groove
26. Distal phalanx [Ungual bone; Coffin bone; Pe
27. Distal part of lateral palmar process

Horse - Digital bones of the hand (Left) (Mediopalmar view)

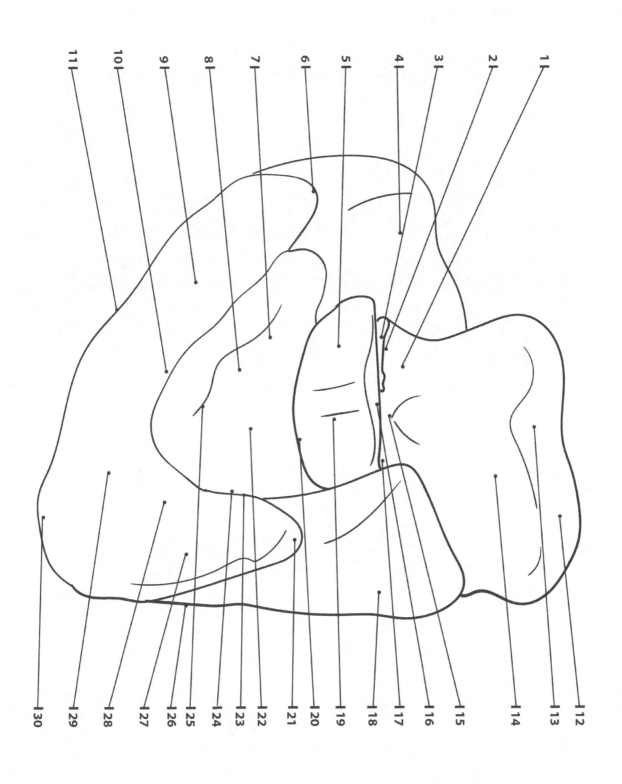

1. Head of middle phalanx
2. Lateral part of distal condyle of middle phal.
3. Distal interphalangeal joint [Coffin joint; DIP j
4. Lateral ungular cartilage
5. Distal sesamoid bone
6. Lateral palmar process
7. Lateral solear groove
8. Lateral solear foramen
9. Cutaneous plane
10. Semilunar line
11. Solar border
12. Base of middle phalanx
13. Flexor tuberosity
14. Middle phalanx [Short pastern bone]
15. Sagittal groove of middle phalanx
16. Proximal border
17. Medial part of distal condyle of middle phal
18. Medial ungular cartilage
19. Flexor surface
20. Distal border
21. Medial palmar process
22. Flexor surface
23. Medial solear groove
24. Medial solear foramen
25. Solar canal
26. Parietal surface
27. Distal phalanx [Ungual bone; Coffin bone; Pez
28. Semilunar sinus
29. Solar surface
30. Notch of solear border

Horse - Bones of the pelvic limb (Left) (Lateral view)

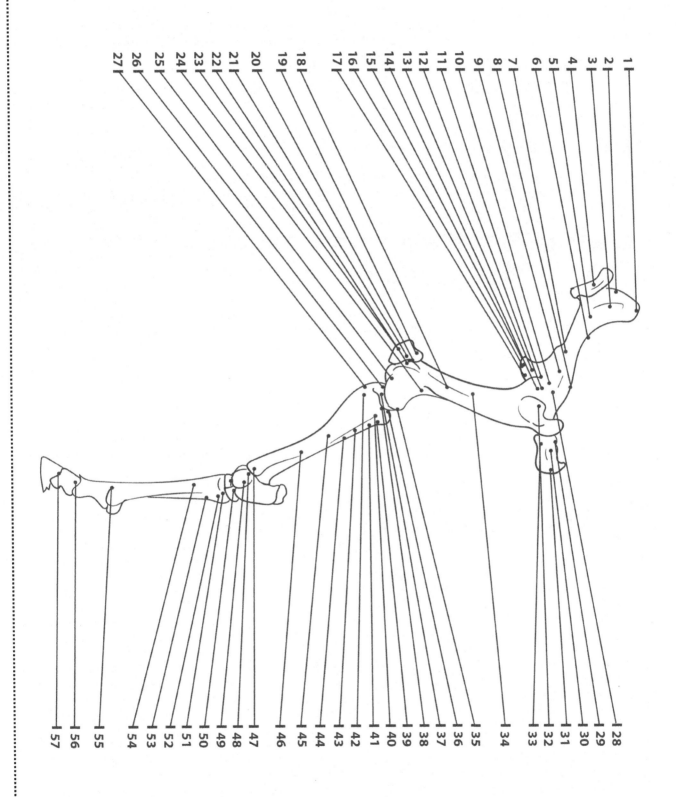

Horse - Bones of the pelvic limb (Left) (Lateral view)

1. Sacral tuberosity
2. Iliac crest
3. Ala of ilium; Wing of ilium
4. Coxal tuberosity
5. Ilium
6. Greater sciatic notch
7. Coxal bone
8. Ischial spine
9. Body of ilium
10. Acetabular margin
11. Hip joint
12. Head of femur
13. Body of pubis
14. Neck of femur
15. Iliopubic eminence
16. Pubis
17. Cranial ramus of pubic bone
18. Thigh bone [Femur]
19. Medial ridge of trochlea of femur
20. Median groove of trochlea of femur
21. Patellofemoral joint
22. Patella
23. Lateral ridge of trochlea of femur
24. Supracondylar fossa
25. Extensor fossa
26. Intercondylar eminence
27. Tibial tuberosity
28. Acetabulum
29. Lesser sciatic notch
30. Ischiatic table
31. Ischial tuberosity
32. Greater trochanter
33. Ischium
34. Body [Shaft] of femur
35. Lateral condyle
36. Femorotibial joint
37. Proximal articular surface
38. Lateral condyle
39. Head of fibula
40. Proximal tibiofibular joint
41. Neck of fibula
42. Extensor groove
43. Body [Shaft] of fibula
44. Fibula
45. Body [Shaft] of tibia
46. Tibia
47. Lateral malleolus
48. Tarsocrural joint
49. Talus
50. Intertarsal joints
51. Tarsometatarsal joints
52. Intermetatarsal joints
53. Metatarsal IV
54. Metatarsal III
55. Metatarsophalangeal joints
56. Proximal interphalangeal joint
57. Distal interphalangeal joint

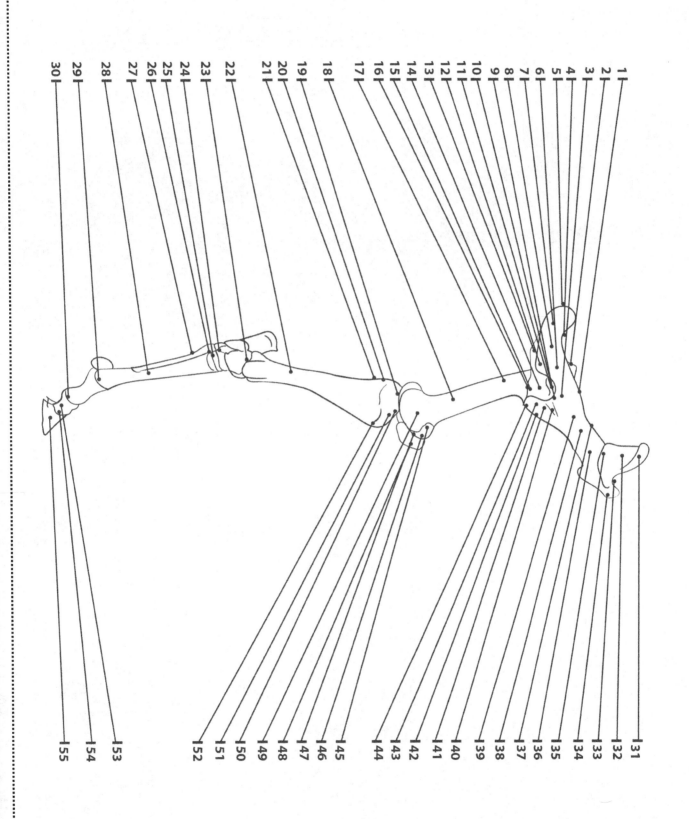

Horse - Bones of the pelvic limb (Left) (Medial view)

1. Ischial spine
2. Greater trochanter
3. Body of ilium
4. Lesser sciatic notch
5. Ischial tuberosity
6. Body of ischium
7. Ischiatic table
8. Ischium
9. Body of pubis
10. Acetabulum
11. Hip joint
12. Ramus of ischium
13. Symphysial surface of ischium
14. Obturator foramen
15. Caudal ramus of pubic bone
16. Symphysial surface of pubis
17. Lesser trochanter
18. Thigh bone [Femur]
19. Femorotibial joint
20. Proximal tibiofibular joint
21. Fibula
22. Tibia
23. Tarsocrural joint
24. Intertarsal joints
25. Tarsometatarsal joints
26. Intermetatarsal joints
27. Metatarsal II
28. Metatarsal III
29. Metatarsophalangeal joints
30. Proximal interphalangeal joint
31. Sacral tuberosity
32. Iliac tuberosity
33. Iliac crest
34. Coxal tuberosity
35. Auricular surface
36. Ala of ilium; Wing of ilium
37. Greater sciatic notch
38. Ilium
39. Coxal bone
40. Obturator groove
41. Pubis
42. Iliopubic eminence
43. Cranial ramus of pubic bone
44. Pecten pubis
45. Tubercle of trochlea of femur
46. Medial ridge of trochlea of femur
47. Patella
48. Patellofemoral joint
49. Medial epicondyle
50. Intercondylar eminence
51. Proximal articular surface
52. Tibial tuberosity
53. Middle phalanx [Short pastern bone]
54. Distal interphalangeal joint
55. Distal phalanx [Ungual bone;Coffin bone; Pedal bone]

Horse - Coxal bone (Left) (Lateral view)

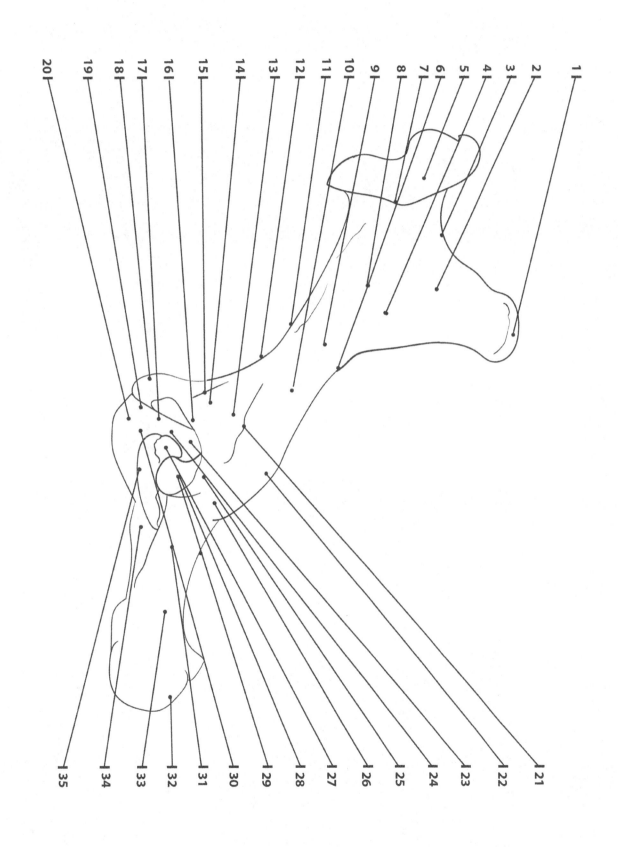

Horse - Coxal bone (Left) (Lateral view)

1. Sacral tuberosity
2. Gluteal surface
3. lliac crest
4. Accessory gluteal line
5. Coxal tuberosity
6. Greater sciatic notch
7. Outer lip
8. Ala of ilium; Wing of ilium
9. Ilium
10. Coxal bone
11. Tubercle for minor psoas
12. Arcuate line
13. Body of ilium
14. Lateral aera of recti femoris
15. Medial area of recti femoris
16. Acetabular margin
17. Body of pubis
18. lliopubic eminence
19. Groove for accessory ligament of femur
20. Cranial ramus of pubic bone
21. Caudal gluteal line
22. Ischial spine
23. Acetabular fossa
24. Acetabular notch
25. Acetabulum
26. Body of ischium
27. Obturator foramen
28. Lunate surface
29. Lesser sciatic notch
30. Pubis
31. Ischium
32. Ischial tuberosity
33. Ischiatic table
34. Ramus of ischium
35. Caudal ramus of pubic bone

Horse - Coxal bone (Left) (Medial view)

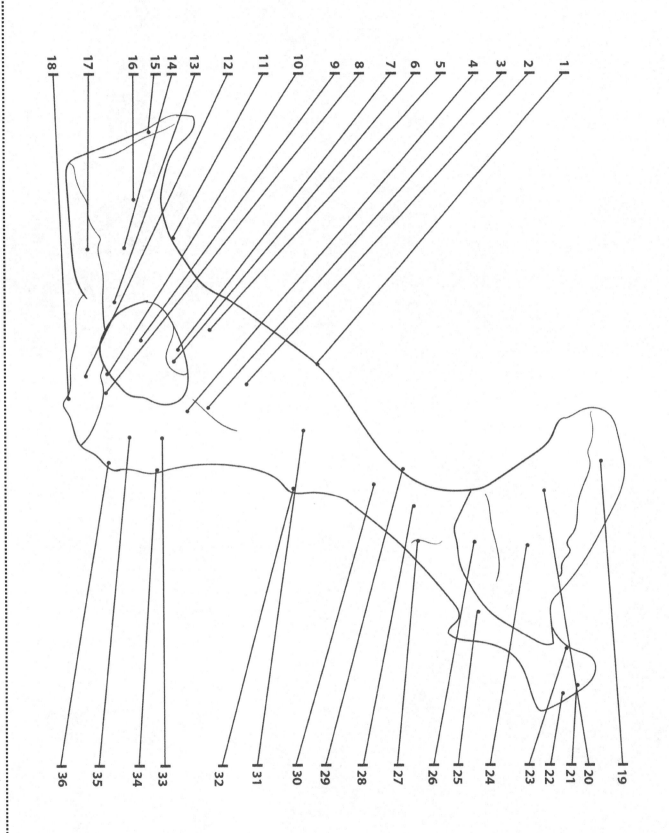

Horse - Coxal bone (Left) (Medial view)

1. Ischial spine
2. Body of ilium
3. Obturator groove
4. Body of pubis
5. Body of ischium
6. Acetabular margin
7. Acetabulum
8. Dorsal pubic tubercle
9. Obturator foramen
10. Caudal ramus of pubic bone
11. Lesser sciatic notch
12. Symphysial surface of pubis
13. Ramus of ischium
14. Ischium
15. Ischial tuberosity
16. Ischiatic table
17. Symphysial surface of ischium
18. Ventral pubic tubercle
19. Sacral tuberosity
20. lliac tuberosity
21. Coxal tuberosity
22. Inner lip
23. lliac crest
24. Sacropelvic surface
25. lliac surface
26. Auricular surface
27. Arcuate line
28. Ala of ilium; Wing of lium
29. Greater sciatic notch
30. lium
31. Coxal bone
32. Tubercle for minor psoas
33. Pubis
34. lliopubic eminence
35. Cranial ramus of pubic bone
36. Pecten pubis

Horse - Girdle of pelvic limb (Cranial view)

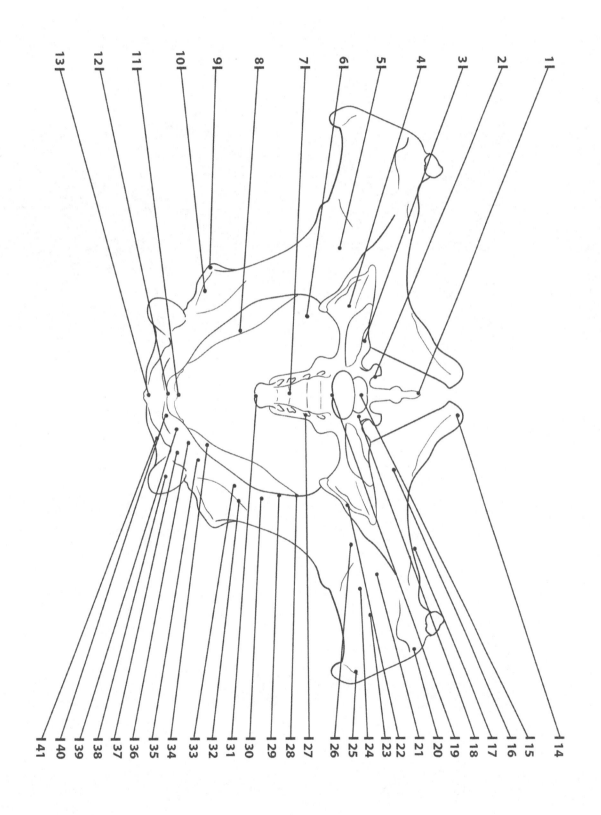

Horse - Girdle of pelvic limb (Cranial view)

1. Median sacral crest
2. Cranial articular process
3. Lateral part of sacrum
4. Ala; Wing of sacrum
5. Coxal bone
6. Pelvic cavity
7. Transverse lines
8. Ischial spine
9. Acetabular margin
10. Acetabulum
11. Dorsal pubic tubercle
12. Pelvic symphysis
13. Ventral pubic tubercle

14. Sacral tuberosity
15. Sacral canal
16. Iliac tuberosity
17. Iliac crest
18. Sacrum [Sacral vertebrae]
19. Promontory
20. Coxal tuberosity
21. Sacropelvic surface
22. Sacroiliac joint
23. Iliac surface
24. Ilium
25. Inner lip
26. Ala of ilium; Wing of ilium
27. Ventral sacral foramina
28. Arcuate line
29. Tubercle for minor psoas
30. Body of ilium
31. Apex of sacrum
32. Lateral aera of recti femoris
33. Medial area of recti femoris
34. Body of ischium
35. Body of pubis
36. Pubis
37. Iliopubic eminence
38. Ischium
39. Cranial ramus of pubic bone
40. Pecten pubis
41. Ischiatic table

Horse - Coxal bone (Cranial view)

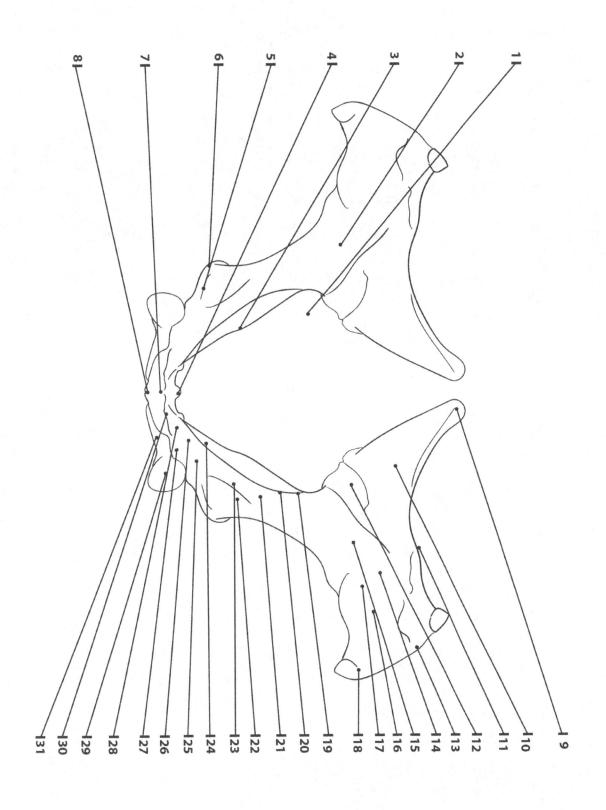

Horse - Coxal bone (Cranial view)

1. Pelvic cavity
2. Coxal bone
3. Ischial spine
4. Dorsal pubic tubercle
5. Acetabulum
6. Acetabular margin
7. Pubic symphysis (Pelvic symphysis)
8. Ventral pubic tubercle
9. Sacral tuberosity
10. lliac tuberosity
11. lliac crest
12. Auricular surface
13. Coxal tuberosity
14. Sacropelvic surface
15. Ala of ilium; Wing of ilium
16. lliac surface
17. lium
18. Inner lip
19. Arcuate line
20. Tubercle for minor psoas
21. Body of ilium
22. Lateral aera of recti femoris
23. Medial area of recti femoris
24. Body of ischium
25. Body of pubis
26. Pubis
27. lliopubic eminence
28. Cranial ramus of pubic bone
29. Ischium
30. Pecten pubis
31. Ischiatic Table

Horse - Coxal bone (Caudal view)

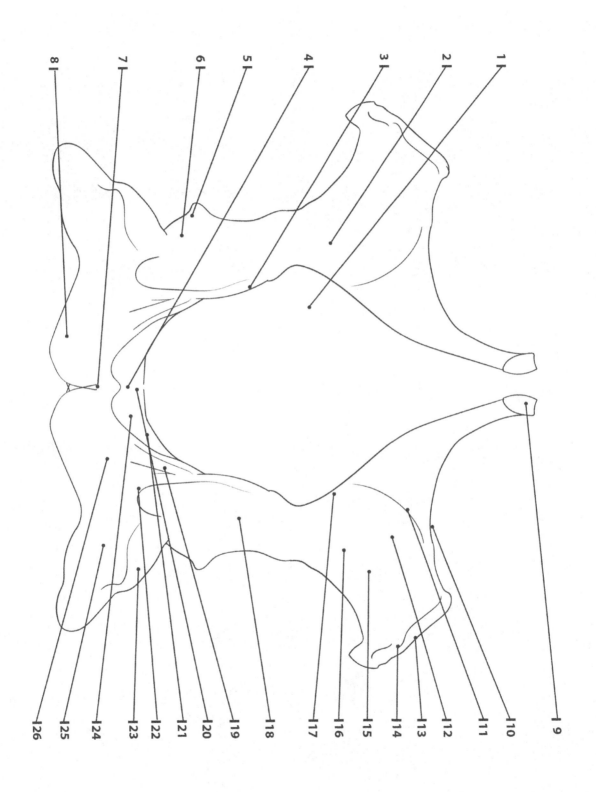

Horse - Coxal bone (Caudal view)

1. Pelvic cavity
2. Coxal bone
3. Ischial spine
4. Pubic symphysis (Pelvic symphysis)
5. Acetabular margin
6. Acetabulum
7. Ischiadic symphysis (Pelvic symphysis)
8. Ischial arch|

9. Sacral tuberosity
10. Iliac crest
11. Accessory gluteal line
12. Ala of ilium; Wing of ilium
13. Coxal tuberosity
14. Outer lip
15. Gluteal surface
16. Ilium
17. Greater sciatic notch
18. Body of ilium
19. Body of ischium
20. Dorsal pubic tubercle
21. Pubis
22. Lesser sciatic notch
23. Ischial tuberosity
24. Cranial ramus of pubic bone
25. Ischium
26. Ischiatic table

Horse - Coxal bone (Dorsal view)

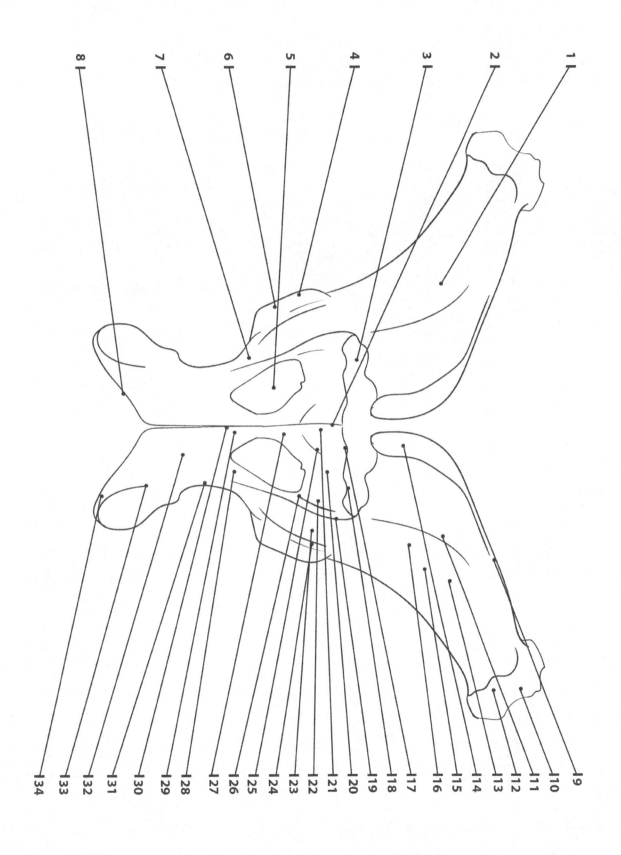

Horse - Coxal bone (Dorsal view)

1. Coxal bone
2. Pubic symphysis (Pelvic symphysis)
3. Pelvic cavity
4. Acetabular margin
5. Obturator foramen
6. Acetabulum
7. Ischial spine
8. Ischial arch
9. Iliac crest
10. Coxal tuberosity
11. Accessory gluteal line
12. Outer lip
13. Ala of ilium; Wing of ilium
14. Sacral tuberosity
15. Gluteal surface
16. Ilium
17. Pecten pubis
18. Iliopubic eminence
19. Greater sciatic notch
20. Cranial ramus of pubic bone
21. Dorsal pubic tubercle
22. Body of pubis
23. Body of ilium
24. Caudal gluteal line
25. Pubis
26. Obturator groove
27. Caudal ramus of pubic bone
28. Body of ischium
29. Ramus of ischium
30. Ischiadic symphysis (Pelvic symphysis)
31. Lesser sciatic notch
32. Ischiatic table
33. Ischium
34. Ischial tuberosity

Horse - Coxal bone (Ventral view)

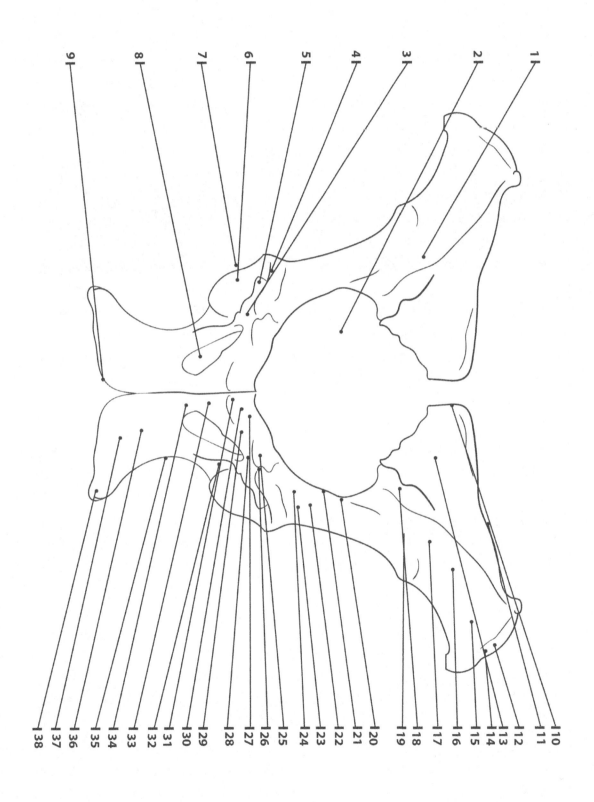

Horse - Coxal bone (Ventral view)

1. Coxal bone
2. Pelvic cavity
3. Acetabular notch
4. Acetabular margin
5. Acetabular fossa
6. Lunate surface
7. Acetabulum
8. Obturator foramen
9. Ischial arch
10. Sacral tuberosity
11. lliac crest
12. Coxal tuberosity
13. lliac tuberosity
14. Inner lip
15. lliac surface
16. Sacropelvic surface
17. Ala of ilium; Wing of ilium
18. Auricular surface
19. lium
20. Arcuate line
21. Tubercle for minor psoas
22. Body of ilium
23. Lateral aera of recti femoris
24. Medial area of recti femoris
25. lliopubic eminence
26. Body of pubis
27. Pecten pubis
28. Groove for accessory ligament of femur
29. Cranial ramus of pubic bone
30. Pubis
31. Ventral pubic tubercle
32. Body of ischium
33. Caudal ramus of pubic bone
34. Ramus of ischium
35. Lesser sciatic notch
36. ischiatic table
37. ischium
38. ischial tuberosity

Horse - Pelvis

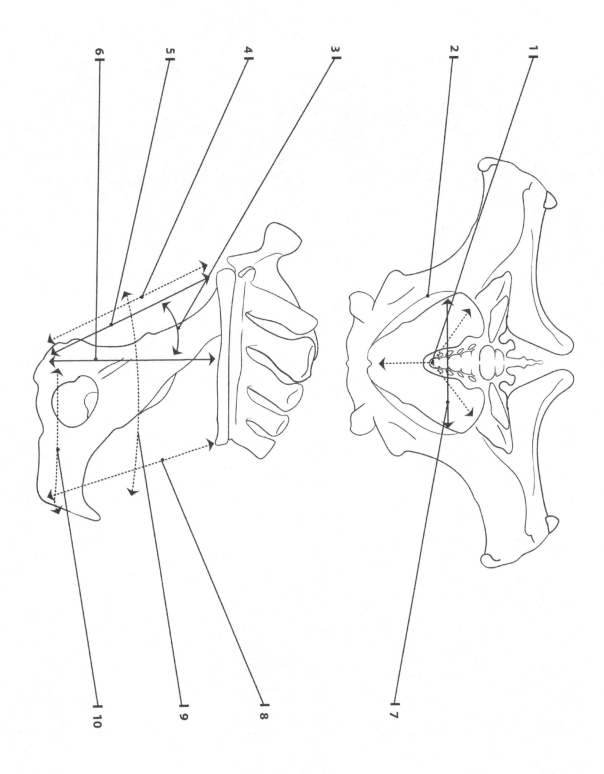

Horse - Pelvis

1. Cranial opening of pelvis
2. Linea terminalis
3. Pelvic inclination
4. Cranial opening of pelvis
5. Conjugate diameter
6. Vertical diameter

7. Transverse diameter
8. Caudal opening of pelvis
9. Axis of pelvis
10. Floor of bony pelvis

Horse - Thigh bone [Femur] (Left) (Lateral view)

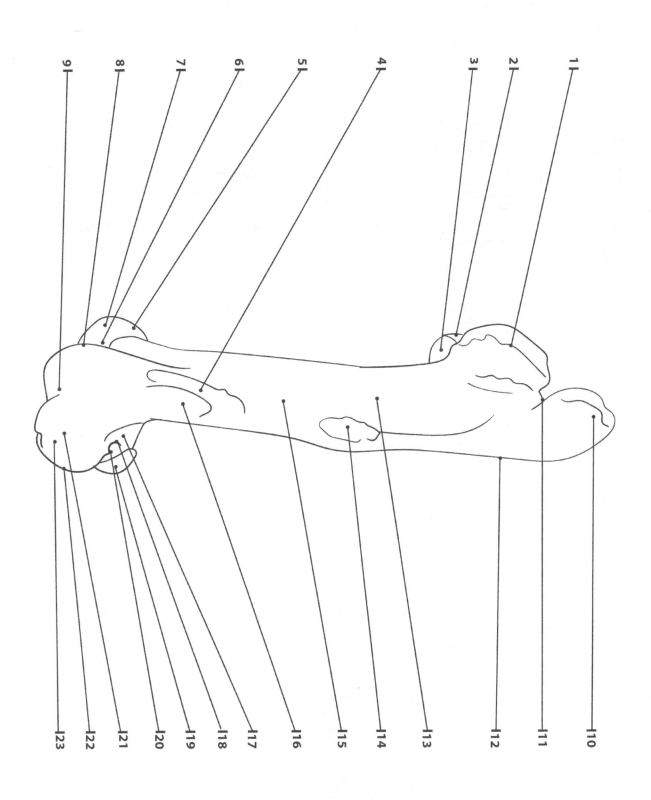

Horse - Thigh bone [Femur] (Left) (Lateral view)

1. Cranial part of greater trochanter
2. Head of femur
3. Neck of femur
4. Lateral supracondylar tub...
5. Tubercle of trochlea of femur
6. Median groove of trochlea of femur
7. Medial ridge of trochlea of femur
8. Lateral ridge of trochlea of femur
9. Extensor fossa
10. Caudal part of greater trochanter
11. Trochanteric notch
12. Intertrochanteric crest
13. Body [Shaft] of femur
14. Third trochanter
15. Thigh bone [Femur]
16. Supracondylar fossa
17. Popliteal surface
18. Intercondylar line
19. Medial condyle
20. Intercondylar fossa
21. Lateral epicondyle:
22. Lateral condyle
23. Fossa for popliteal

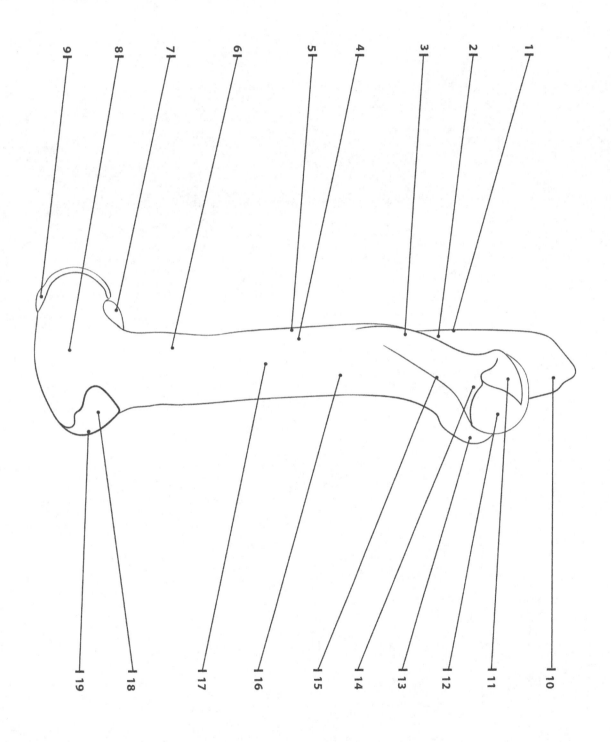

Horse - Thigh bone [Femur] (Left) (Medial view)

1. Intertrochanteric crest
2. Trochanteric fossa
3. Lesser trochanter
4. Medial lip
5. Facies aspera
6. Medial supracondylar tuberosity
7. Lateral condyle
8. Medial epicondyle
9. Medial condyle

10. Caudal part of greater trochanter
11. Fovea for ligament of head
12. Head of femur
13. Cranial part of greater trochanter
14. Neck of femur
15. Intertrochanteric line
16. Body [Shaft] of femur
17. Thigh bone [Femur]
18. Tubercle of trochlea of femur
19. Medial ridge of trochlea of femur

Horse - Thigh bone [Femur] (Left) (Cranial view)

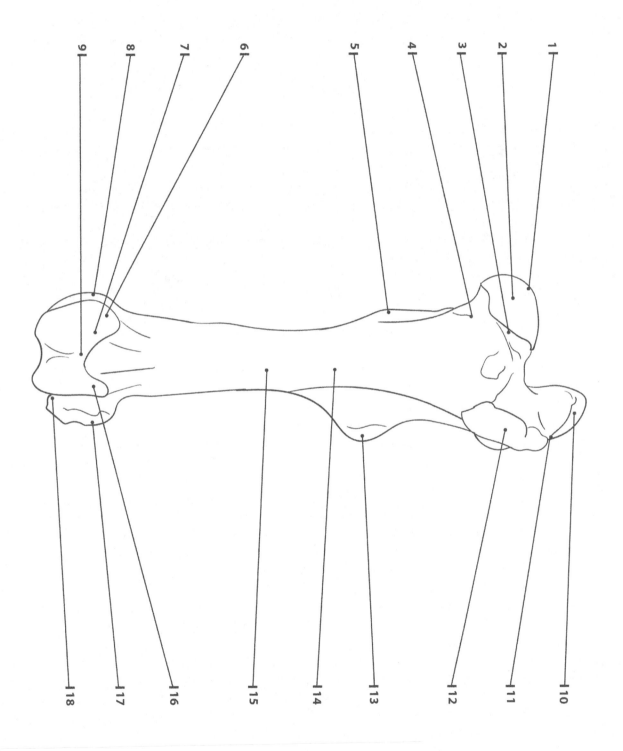

Horse - Thigh bone [Femur] (Left) (Cranial view)

1. Fovea for ligament of head
2. Head of femur
3. Neck of femur
4. Intertrochanteric line
5. Lesser trochanter
6. Tubercle of trochlea of femur
7. Medial ridge of trochlea of femur
8. Medial epicondyle
9. Median groove of trochlea of femur
10. Caudal part of greater trochanter
11. Trochanteric notch
12. Cranial part of greater trochanter
13. Third trochanter
14. Body [Shaft] of femur
15. Thigh bone [Femur]
16. Lateral ridge of trochlea of femur
17. Lateral epicondyle
18. Extensor fossa

Horse - Thigh bone [Femur] (Left) (Caudal view)

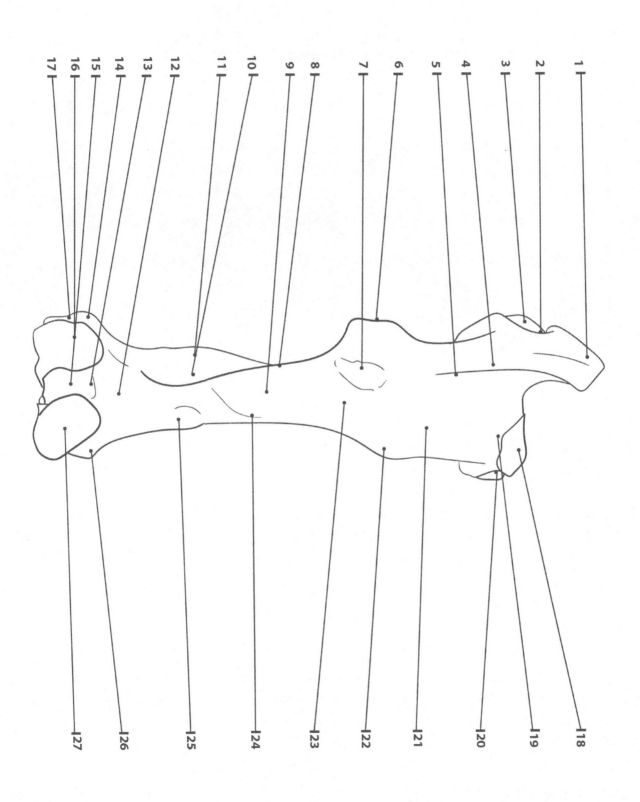

Horse - Thigh bone [Femur] (Left) (Caudal view)

1. Caudal part of greater trochanter
2. Trochanteric notch
3. Cranial part of greater trochanter
4. Intertrochanteric crest
5. Trochanteric fossa
6. Third trochanter
7. Tuberosity of the biceps
8. Lateral lip
9. Facies aspera
10. Supracondylar fossa
11. Lateral supracondylar tuberosity
12. Popliteal surface
13. Intercondylar line
14. Lateral epicondyle
15. Intercondylar fossa
16. Lateral condyle
17. Fossa for popliteal
18. Head of femur
19. Neck of femur
20. Fovea for ligament of head
21. Thigh bone [Femur]
22. Lesser trochanter
23. Body [Shaft] of femur
24. Medial lip
25. Medial supracondylar tuberosity
26. Medial epicondyle
27. Medial condyle

Horse - Thigh bone [Femur] (Left) (Proximal view)

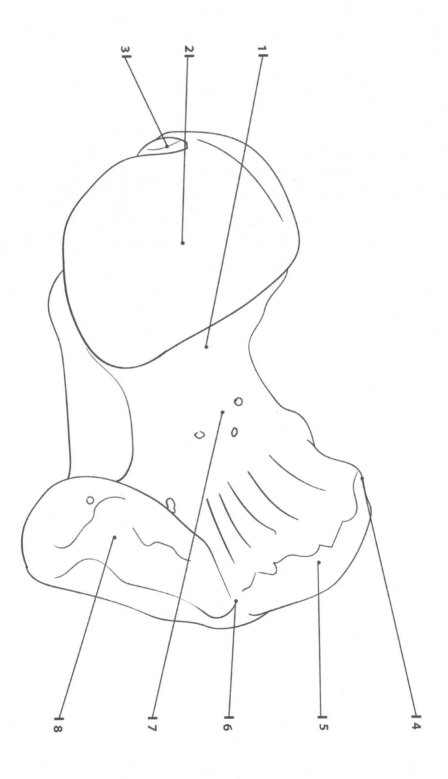

Horse - Thigh bone [Femur] (Left) (Proximal view)

1. Neck of femur
2. Head of femur
3. Fovea for ligament of head

4. Intertrochanteric crest
5. Caudal part of greater trochanter
6. Trochanteric notch
7. Thigh bone [Femur]
8. Cranial part of greater trochanter

Horse - Thigh bone [Femur] (Left) (Distal view)

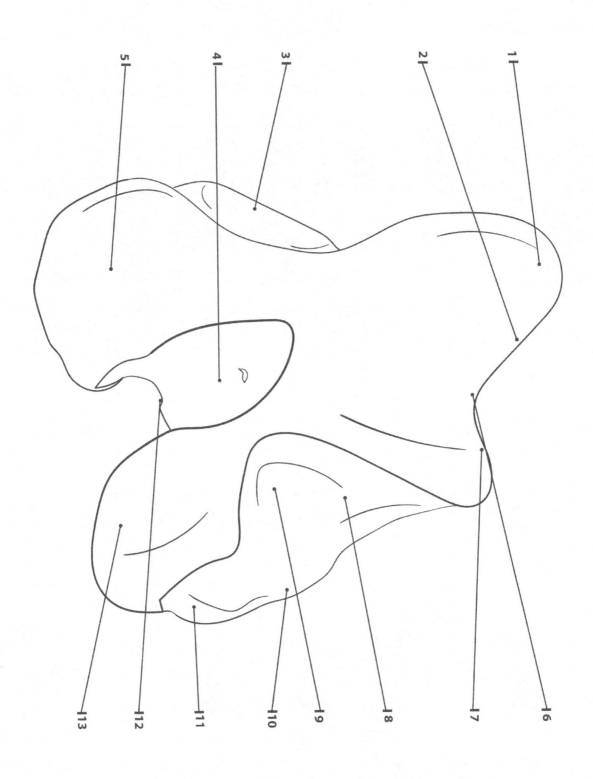

Horse - Thigh bone [Femur] (Left) (Distal view)

1. Tubercle of trochlea of femur
2. Medial ridge of trochlea of femur
3. Medial epicondyle
4. Intercondylar fossa
5. Medial condyle

6. Median groove of trochlea of femur
7. Lateral ridge of trochlea of femur
8. Thigh bone [Femur]
9. Extensor fossa
10. Lateral epicondyle
11. Fossa for popliteal
12. Intercondylar line
13. Lateral condyle

Horse - Patella (Left) (Cranial view)

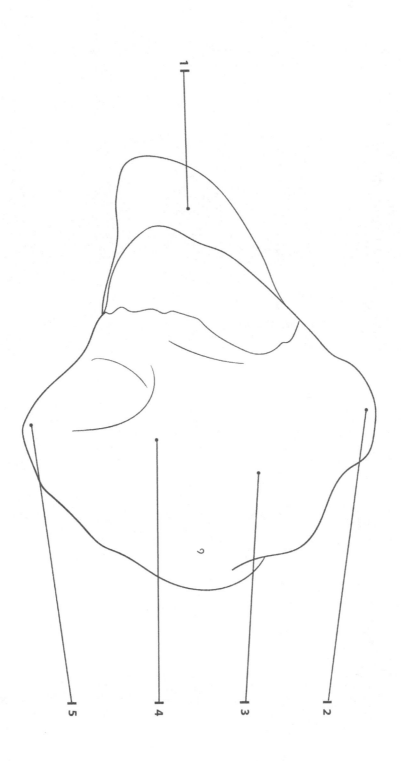

Horse - Patella (Left) (Cranial view)

1. Cartilaginous process

2. Base of patella
3. Cranial surface
4. Patella
5. Apex of patella

Horse - Patella (Left) (Caudal view)

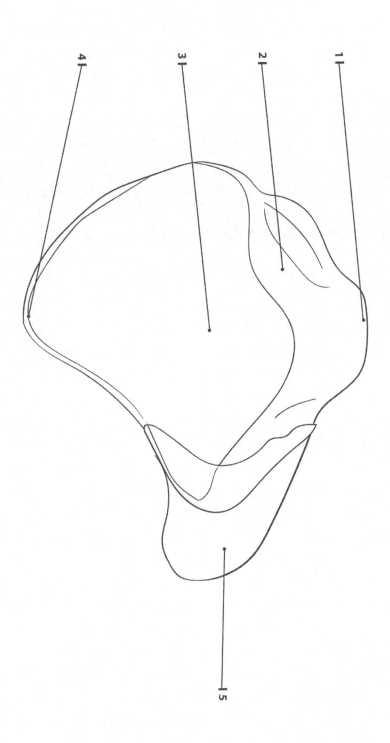

1.Base of patella

2.Patella

3.Articular surface

4.Apex of patella

5.Cartilaginous process

Horse - Tibia / Fibula (Left) (Lateral view)

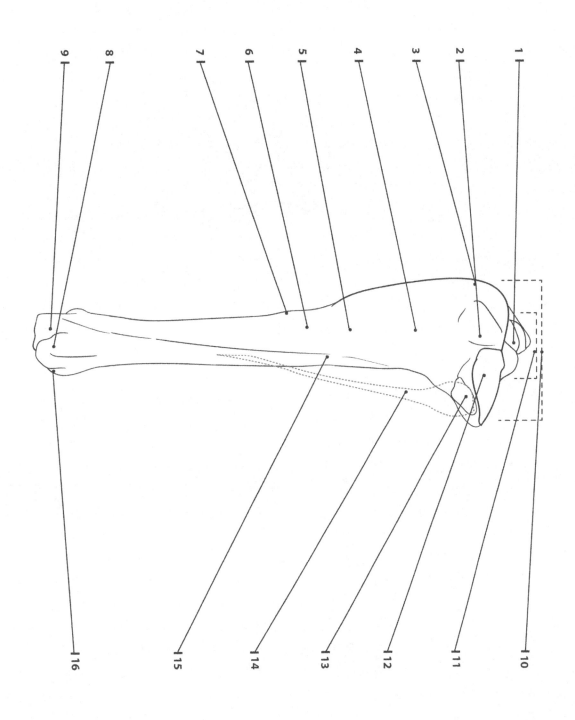

Horse - Tibia / Fibula (Left) (Lateral view)

1. Lateral intercondylar tubercle
2. Extensor groove
3. Tibial tuberosity
4. Tibia
5. Body [Shaft] of tibia
6. Lateral surface
7. Cranial border
8. Malleolar groove
9. Lateral malleolus
10. Proximal articular surface
11. Intercondylar eminence
12. Lateral condyle
13. Fibular articular facet
14. Fibula
15. Lateral margin [Inteosseous margin]
16. Cochlea of tibia

Horse - Tibia / Fibula (Left) (Medial view)

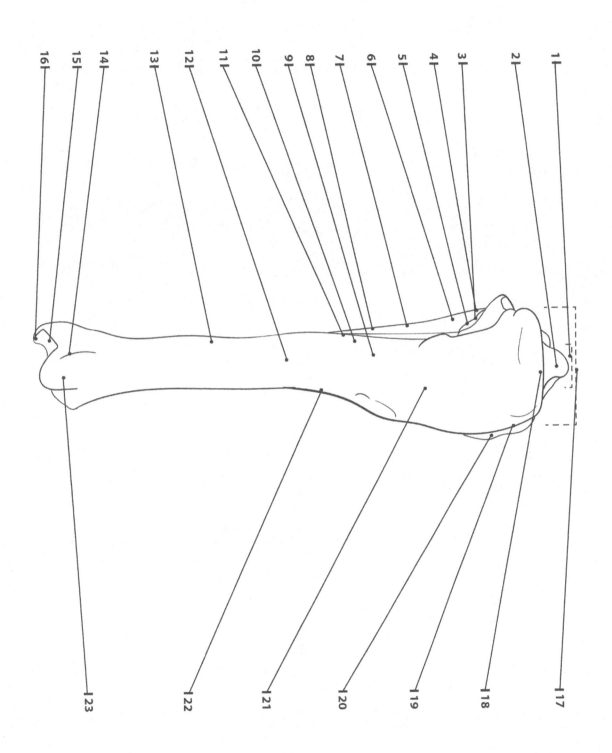

Horse - Tibia / Fibula (Left) (Medial view)

1. Intercondylar eminence
2. Medial intercondylar tubercle
3. Articular facet of head of fibula
4. Head of fibula
5. Proximal tibiofibular joint
6. Neck of fibula
7. Body [Shaft] of fibula
8. Fibula
9. Body [Shaft] of tibia
10. Line of popliteus muscle
11. Caudal surface
12. Tibia
13. Medial margin
14. Malleolar groove
15. Cochlea of tibia
16. Intermediate ridge of tibial cochlea

17. Proximal articular surface
18. Medial condyle
19. Groove of tibial tuberosity
20. Tibial tuberosity
21. Medial surface
22. Cranial border
23. Medial malleolus

Horse-Tibia / Fibula (Left) (Cranial view)

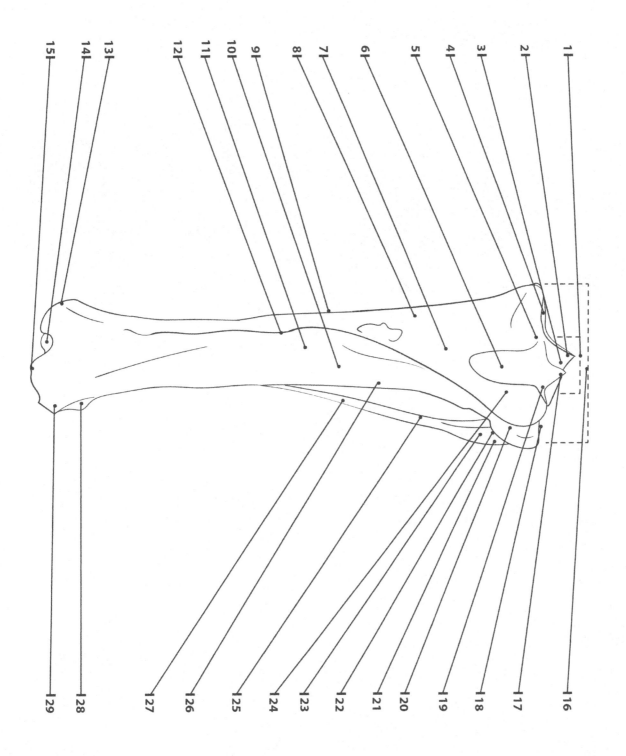

Horse-Tibia / Fibula (Left) (Cranial view)

1. Intercondylar eminence
2. Medial intercondylar tubercle
3. Central intercondylar area
4. Medial condyle
5. Cranial intercondylar area
6. Groove of tibial tuberosity
7. Tibia
8. Medial surface
9. Medial margin
10. Lateral surface
11. Body [Shaft] of tibia
12. Cranial border
13. Medial malleolus
14. Cochlea of tibia
15. Intermediate ridge of tibial cochlea
16. Proximal articular surface
17. Lateral intercondylar tubercle
18. Lateral condyle
19. Cranial intercondylar area
20. Extensor groove
21. Head of fibula
22. Proximal tibiofibular joint
23. Neck of fibula
24. Tibial tuberosity
25. Body [Shaft] of fibula
26. Lateral margin [Inteosseous margin]
27. Fibula
28. Malleolar groove
29. Lateral malleolus

Horse - Tibia / Fibula (Left) (Caudal view)

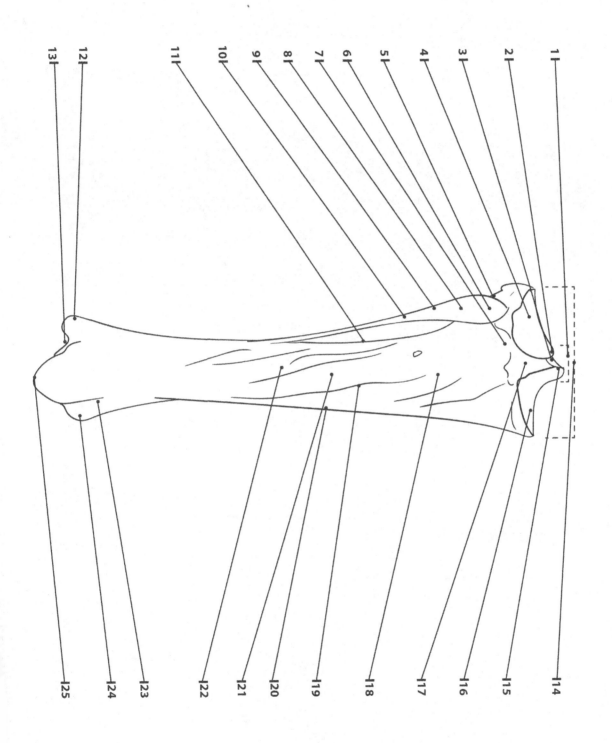

Horse - Tibia / Fibula (Left) (Caudal view)

1. Intercondylar eminence
2. Lateral intercondylar tubercle
3. Central intercondylar area
4. Lateral condyle
5. Proximal tibiofibular joint
6. Head of fibula
7. Popliteal notch
8. Neck of fibula
9. Fibula
10. Body [Shaft] of fibula
11. Lateral margin[Inteosseous margin]
12. Lateral malleolus
13. Cochlea of tibia
14. Proximal articular surface
15. Medial intercondylar tubercle
16. Medial condyle
17. Caudal intercondylar area
18. Body [Shaft] of tibia
19. Line of popliteus muscle
20. Medial margin
21. Caudal surface
22. Tibia
23. Malleolar groove
24. Medial malleolus
25. Intermediate ridge-of tibial cochlea

Horse - Tibia (Left) (Proximal view)

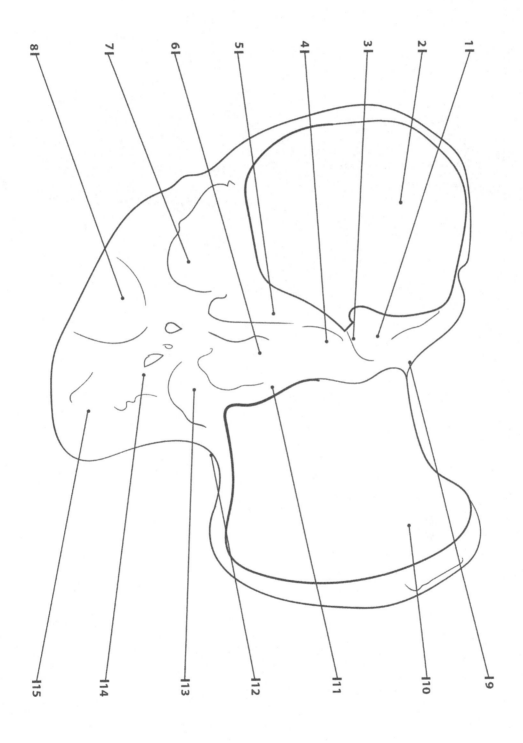

Horse - Tibia (Left) (Proximal view)

1. Caudal intercondylar area
2. Medial condyle
3. Proximal articular surface
4. Intercondylar eminence
5. Medial intercondylar tubercle
6. Central intercondylar area
7. Cranial intercondylar area
8. Groove of tibial tuberosity
9. Popliteal notch
10. Lateral condyle
11. Lateral intercondylar tubercle
12. Extensor groove
13. Cranial intercondylar area
14. Tibia
15. Tibial tuberosity

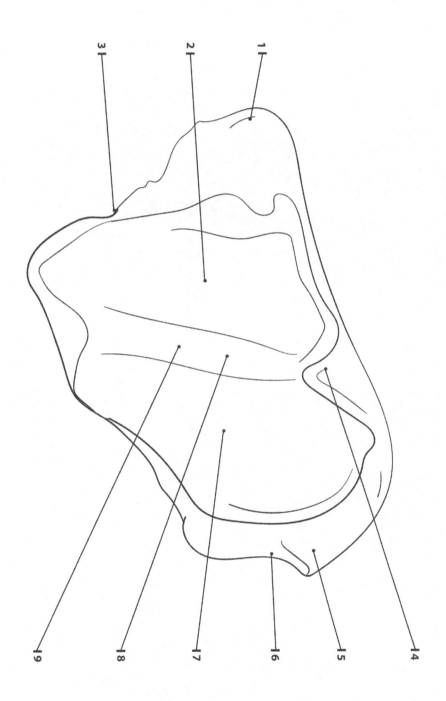

Horse - Tibia (Left) (Distal view)

1. Medial malleolus
2. Medial groove of tibial cochlea
3. Malleolar groove

4. Tibia
5. Lateral malleolus
6. Malleolar groove
7. Lateral groove of tibial cochlea
8. Cochlea of tibia
9. Intermediate ridge of tibial cochlea

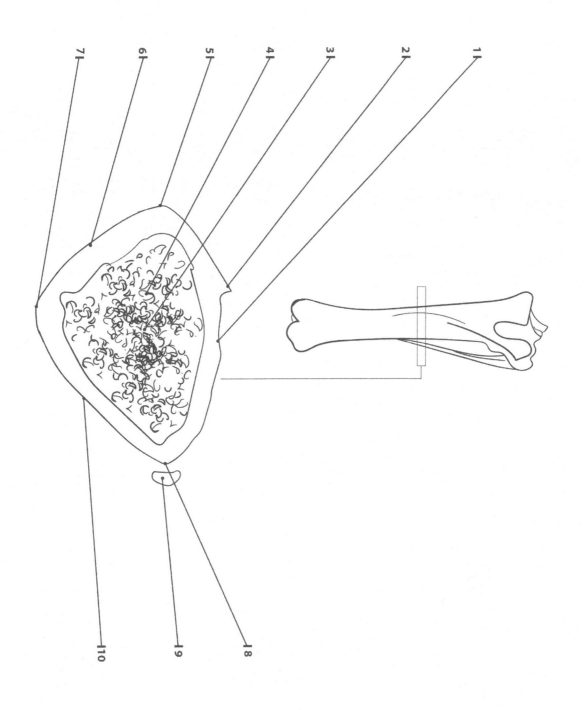

Horse - Tibia / Fibula (Left) (Axial cross section)

1. Caudal surface
2. Line of popliteus muscle
3. Body [Shaft] of tibia
4. Tibia
5. Medial margin
6. Medial surface
7. Cranial border

8. Lateral margin [Inteosseous margin]
9. Fibula
10. Lateral surface

Horse - Tarsus (Left) (Lateral view)

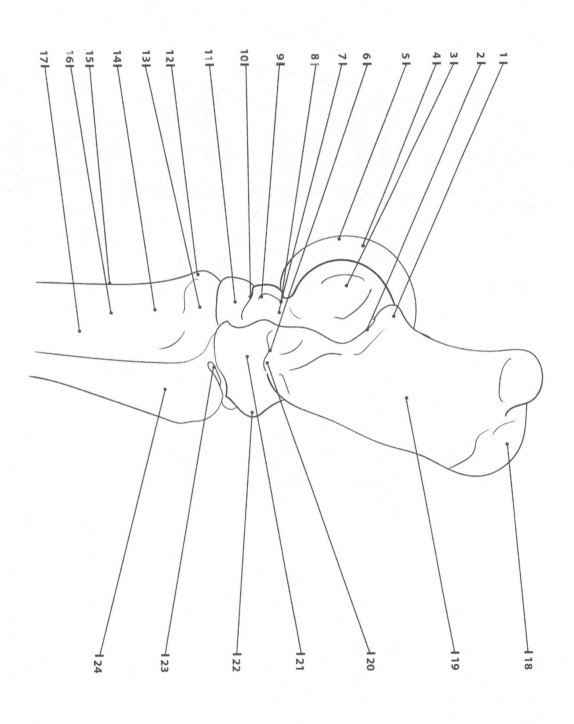

Horse - Tarsus (Left) (Lateral view)

1. Coracoid process
2. Talocalcaneal joint
3. Talus
4. Trochlea of talus
5. Lateral ridge of trochlea tali
6. Articular surface for cuboid
7. Navicular articular surface
8. Talocalcaneocentral joint
9. Central tarsal bone [Navicular bone]
10. Centrodistal joint [Cuneonavicular joint]
11. Tarsal bone III [Lateral cuneiform]
12. Tuberosity of third metatarsal
13. Base
14. Metatarsal III
15. Dorsal surface
16. Shaft; Body
17. Lateral surface
18. Calcaneal tuberosity
19. Caleaneus
20. Calcaneoquartal joint [Calcaneocuboid joint]
21. Tarsal bone IV [Cuboid]
22. Tuberosity of tarsal bone IV
23. Intermetatarsal joints
24. Metatarsal IV

Horse - Tarsus (Left) (Medial view)

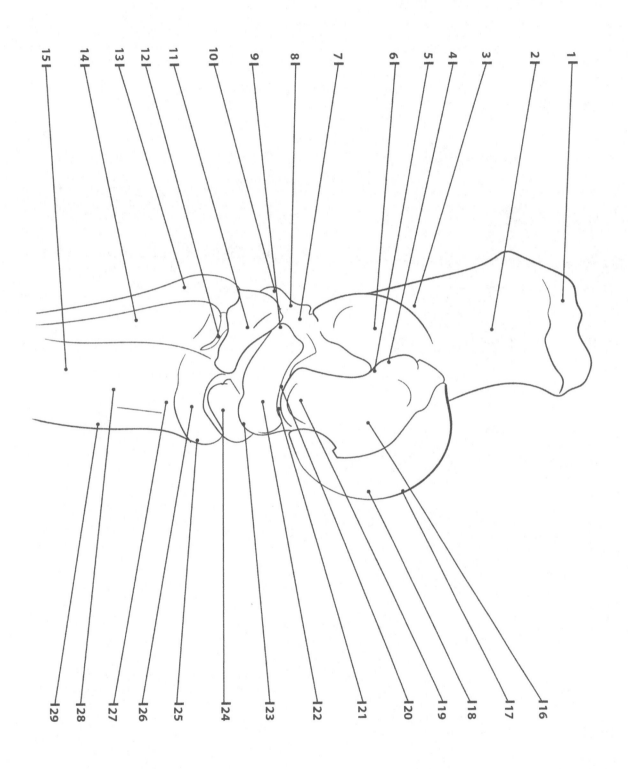

Horse - Tarsus (Left) (Medial view)

1. Calcaneal tuberosity
2. Calcaneus
3. Groove for tendon of lateral digital flexor...
4. Talocalcaneal joint
5. Tarsal sinus
6. Sustentaculum tali;Talar shelf
7. Calcaneoquartaljoint [Calcaneocuboid j...
8. Tarsal bone IV [Cuboid]
9. Plantar tuberosity of central tarsal bone
10. Tuberosity of tarsal bone IV
11. Tarsal bone I and II
12. Intermetatarsal joints
13. Metatarsal IV
14. Metatarsal II
15. Medial surface
16. Talus
17. Medial ridge of trochlea tali
18. Trochlea of talus
19. Tubercle of talus
20. Talocalcaneocentral joint
21. Navicular articular surface
22. Central tarsal bone [Navicular bone]
23. Centrodistal joint [Cuneonavicular joint]
24. Tarsal bone Ill [Lateral cuneiform]
25. Tuberosity of third metatarsal
26. Base
27. Metatarsal III
28. Shaft; Body
29. Dorsal surface

Horse - Tarsus (Left) (Dorsal view)

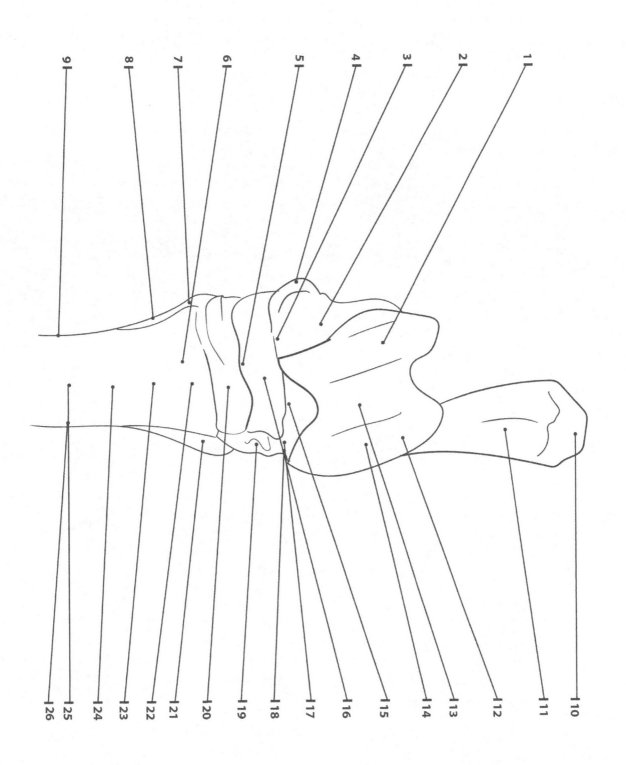

Horse - Tarsus (Left) (Dorsal view)

1. Medial ridge of trochlea tali
2. Talus
3. Talocalcaneocentral joint [Talocalcaneonavi
4. Tubercle of talus
5. Centrodistal joint| [Cuneonavicular joint]
6. Tuberosity of third metatarsal
7. Intermetatarsal joints
8. Metatarsal II
9. Medial surface
10. Calcaneal tuberosity
11. Calcaneus
12. Lateral ridge of trochlea tali
13. Central groove of trochlea of talus
14. Trochlea of talus
15. Navicular articular surface
16. Central tarsal bone [Navicular bone]
17. Articular surface for cuboid
18. Calcaneoquartaljoint [Calcaneocuboid joint]
19. Tarsal bone IV [Cuboid]
20. Tarsal bone III [Lateral cuneiform]
21. Metatarsal IV
22. Base
23. Metatarsal III
24. Shaft; Body
25. Dorsal surface
26. Lateral surface

Horse - Tarsus (Left) (Plantar view)

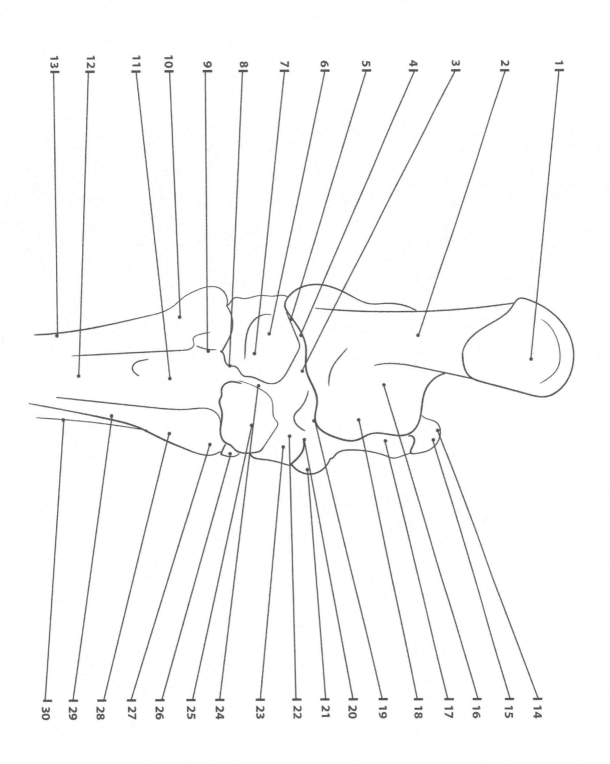

Horse - Tarsus (Left) (Plantar view)

1.Calcaneal tuberosity
2.Calcaneus
3.Tarsal sinus
4.Articular surface for cuboid
5.Calcaneoquartaljoint [Calcaneocuboid joint]
6.Tarsal bone IV [Cuboid]
7.Tuberosity of tarsal bone IV
8.Tarsal canal
9.Intermetatarsal joints
10.Metatarsal IV
11.Metatarsal III
12.Plantar surface
13.Lateral surface|

14. Medial ridge of trochlea tali
15. Trochlea of talus
16. Groove for tendon of lateral digital flexor mus.
17. Talus
18. Sustentaculum tali; Talarshelf
19. Talocalcaneal joint
20. Talocalcaneocentral joint [Talocalcaneonavicular j
21. Tubercle of talus
22. Central tarsal bone [Navicular bone]
23. Plantar tuberosity of central tarsal bone
24. Centrodistal joint [Cuneonavicular joint]
25. Tarsal bone I and II
26. Tarsal bone III [Lateral cuneiform]
27. Base
28. Metatarsal II
29. Shaft; Body
30. Medial Surface

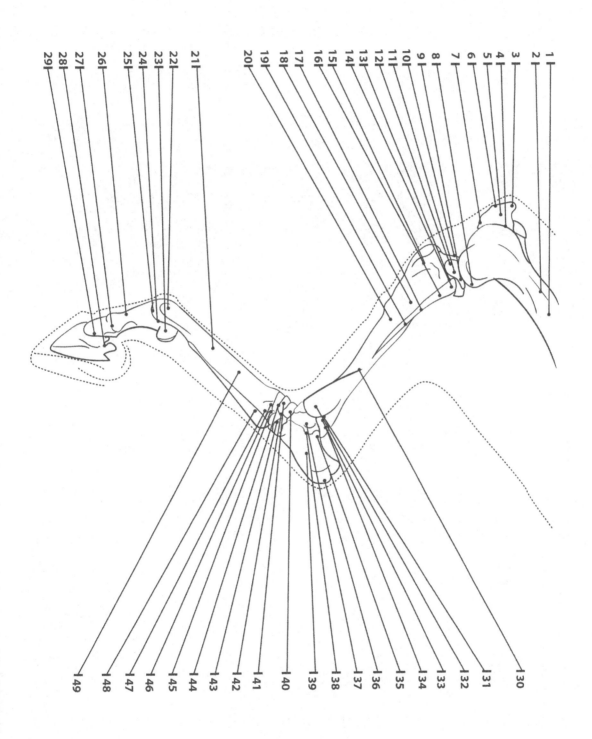

Horse - Leg (Left) (Lateral view)

1.Body [Shaft] of femur
2.Thigh bone [Femur]
3.Base of patella
4.Patellofemoral joint
5.Patella
6.Cranial surface
7.Apex of patella
8.Lateral condyle
9.Femorotibial joint
10.Intercondylar eminence
11.Lateral condyle
12.Proximal articular surface
13.Head of ula
14.Proximal tibiofiular joint
15.Neck of fibula
16.Extensor groove
17.Body [Shaff] of fibula
18.Tibia
19.Fibula
20.Body [Shaft] of tibia
21.Metatarsal III
22.Head
23.Proximal sesamoid bones
24.Lateral plantar eminence
25.Metatarsophalangeal joints
26.Proximal phalanx [Long pastem bone]
27.Proximal interphalangeal joint
28.Distal sesamoid bone
29.Distal interphalangeal joint

30. Lateral margin [Inteosseous margin]
31. Lateral malleolus
32. Malleolar groove
33. Tarsocrural joint
34. Trochlea of talus
35. Coracoid process
36. Calcaneal tuberosity
37. Talus
38. Talocaleaneal joint
39. Calcaneus
40. Central tarsal bone [Navicular bone]
41. Tarsal bone Ill [Lateral cuneiform]
42. Intertarsal joints
43. Tarsal bone IV [Cuboid]
44. Tarsometatarsal joints
45. Tuberosity of third metatarsal
46. Base
47. Intermetatarsal joints
48. Metatarsal IV
49. Shaft; Body